11.00

P9-ECQ-627

Growing Up with Sex

Richard Hettlinger

Growing Up with Sex
A Guide for the Early Teens

New Revised Edition

CONTINUUM · New York

CAMROSE LUTHERAN COLLEGE
LIBRARY

1980
The Continuum Publishing Corporation
815 Second Avenue, New York, NY 10017

Copyright © 1970, 1971; text revision
copyright 1980 by Richard F. Hettlinger.
Illustrations by Frank Price

Printed in the United States of America

No part of this book may be reproduced,
stored in a retrieval system, or transmitted,
in any form or by any means, electronic,
mechanical, photocopying, recording, or
otherwise, without the written permission
of The Continuum Publishing Corporation.

Library of Congress Cataloging in Publication Data
Hettlinger, Richard Frederick.
Growing up with sex.
Bibliography.
SUMMARY: A discussion of sexual development and activity with emphasis on
the emotional aspects.
1. Sex instruction for youth.
2. Adolescence.   3. Sexual ethics.
[1. Sex instruction for youth.
2. Adolescence.   3. Sexual ethics]
I. Price, Frank.   II. Title.
HQ35.H45   1980   613.9'5'088055
80-16016
ISBN 0-8164-0138-1
ISBN 0-8264-0011-6 (pbk.)

Contents

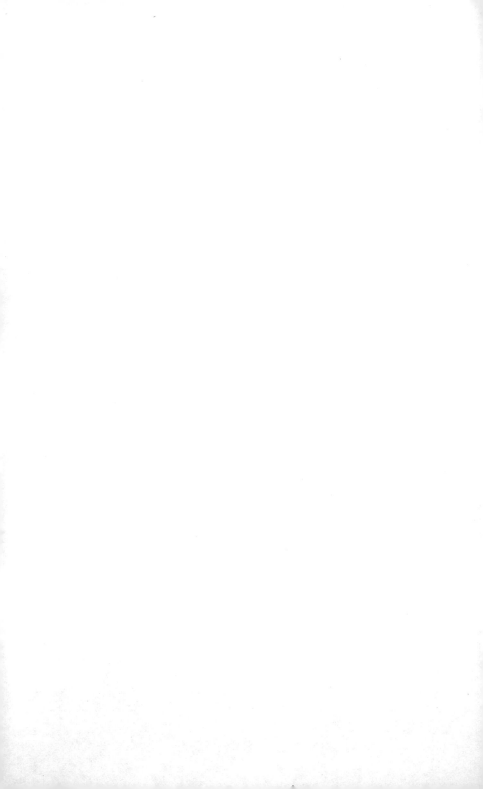

Introduction

Sex can be among the most wonderful and enriching
aspects of life; but it can also be confusing, frustrating
and disappointing—especially when you are somewhere
between childhood and adulthood. The aim of this book
is to give some help to boys and girls anywhere from ten
on, so that the process of growing up with sex will be as
enjoyable and positive as it can be.

You may want accurate information about vaginas and
penises and menstruation and intercourse. You may want
to know how to avoid getting pregnant and how to recognize the diseases passed on by sexual contact. You'll find
that kind of factual material in chapters 1 and 8, and
you'll find a definition of the important words on pages
120 to 129.

You may think you know the basic facts (though the
chances are you're wrong about that) and you may be
more interested in questions like: "Should we go all the
way?" or "How does someone know he's gay?" I hope this
book will help you with these more difficult questions. It's
about the whole complicated process of growing up as a
girl or a boy, becoming a man or a woman, and learning
how to make the most of your relationships with various
groups of people—your family, your peers, society as a

1

whole—as well as those you have sex with in the narrower sense of that word.

(Sex plays a central part in the growth of the human personality, and if it is regarded merely as a way of having fun (or merely as a way of having babies) something of human maturity is missed. Sex isn't something a person *does* at certain times, but is an inseparable part of life from the moment you first breathe—and even before. When the sperm penetrates the ovum to start the process of growth that leads to birth nine months later, the question of the baby's sex is already settled. If the father happens to contribute an X cell with male (Y) chromosomes it is a boy; if his sperm contains female (X) chromosomes it is a girl. Which it is depends on the pure chance of which sperm among many thousands succeeds in entering the ovum; however, it affects not only the individual's physical make-up but his or her whole way of life from birth on. All of us have to grow up with sex as male or female. The question sometimes asked, "Is it wrong to want sex?" is about as sensible as asking, "Is it wrong to want food?" Whether it is right or wrong to engage in particular sex *acts*—or rather, when it is stupid and when it is sensible to do so—are questions we shall discuss. But I must begin by emphasizing that sex is something we all *have,* whether we happen to want it or not.(One of the most unfortunate but common errors is to use the word *sex* as the equivalent of *intercourse.* When people hear that a couple are having "sexual relations" they usually assume that they are sleeping together; but any boy and girl who know each other more than at a distance (and sometimes even then) have a sexual relationship of some kind. All the degrees of intimacy from holding hands or a goodnight kiss to intercourse itself are part of sex, and our relationships to many people with whom we never have any physical contact are basically sexual.

(So growing up with sex cannot be explained in simple,

objective terms. It is possible, of course, to describe what actually happens to the sexual organs when intercourse takes place—though, since there's nothing really comparable to the experience of orgasm, it can't be adequately described in words even as a physical process. But you can't have intercourse on your own, and what it is "actually like" will depend on your attitude to the other person and the circumstances in which you engage in sexual intimacy. This is particularly true for the girl, whose ability to enjoy heavy petting or intercourse is closely tied up with her feelings about the boy and his relationship to her.

Because sex is so important and complex there are limits to what a book like this can do to help you understand it. No book can take the place of people in sex education. Unfortunately most adolescents learn more about sex from what adults *don't* tell them than from what they do. Many find that their parents, who are normally delighted to help with information on any subject, suddenly clam up or show embarrassment over questions about reproduction or the genitals. They get the feeling that adolescent interest in sex is vaguely undesirable or disapproved of by grown-ups; and as a result they often have difficulty talking about their problems with the people who could help most.

It may be worth remembering that your parents had even less help when they were young. Although sexual *behavior* was not all that different a generation ago, open discussion of the subject is still relatively new. Many parents don't really know much about the subject, and therefore find it difficult to discuss or explain sexual development. But there is a more fundamental problem which even the best-informed parent cannot overcome. The subject of sex is never a purely academic, objective matter for discussion between parent and child. It is rather like a father teaching his son to drive an automobile: personal relationships, anxieties, emotional responses all affect the lesson and it usually ends in failure. Almost everyone finds it better to have the job done by someone who is not personally involved with the pupil. While it's certainly desirable that parents should establish healthy and open attitudes to sex by answering questions without embarrassment, it may be best if the details are taught in school or through a book. How children and adolescents *act* in the light of the information will still be influenced by parental standards—just as standards of driving are influenced by whether your father is ruthless or considerate behind the wheel—but don't blame your parents if they find it difficult to provide you with all the help you'd like from them.

This book may not offer you all you'd like either. If you're looking for ready-made answers about how you should behave, you won't find them here. I can only offer you some help: I can't relieve you of the responsibility for the decisions you, as an individual person, will have to make about your own sexuality. I don't believe that anyone—parents, church, or society—can usefully lay down simple rules for everyone to live by. I don't believe most teenagers would, or should accept such rules without question. The best I can do is to present various points of view with fairness, without hiding my own convictions about the most satisfying approach to growing up with sex.

Whether my way of thinking (which, of course, owes a great deal to other writers and to discussions with teenagers) will make sense to you or not, I cannot tell. I hope it does; on the whole, however, I'm not really interested in having you agree with me. I shall be well satisfied if I can help you to steer your way successfully through the confusing tensions of sexual desires and personal ideals that are unavoidable in adolescence. What matters is that you eventually work out a conscious pattern of life and behavior that honestly reflects the distinctive person you are. You are a unique human being, with the freedom to discover what values can best help to develop your potential as a healthy, mature, and happy man or woman. Don't run the risk of disease or pregnancy or forced marriage because of ignorance. Don't just drift through life without coherence or dignity, conforming thoughtlessly to the sexual rules of adult society *or* to the standards of your peers. Don't allow your natural desire for sexual experience and pleasure to rob you of the privilege of being a human being with responsibility for people you know and love.

1 · The Way We Are: Sex Organs and Reproduction

This chapter describes the male and female sex organs, and the process of fertilization and birth. If you've read anything on the subject before, or had an elementary course on sex education at school or elsewhere you will probably be inclined to skip the chapter at this point. That's all right, but don't forget that most people (including adults) have many mistaken ideas about the human body and how it works. So when you're faced with the actual situation of engaging in sexual intercourse or becoming a parent take the trouble to brush up on your knowledge. Better still, do it now and read on, even though you may think you know it all. I bet there will be some things you didn't know before.

The Male Sex Organs

The penis is composed of spongy tissue normally limp and pliable, with a soft tip (the glans) that is reddish-purple in color. Running through its center is a narrow tube (the urethra) which leads to an opening at the end of the glans (the meatus). At birth the glans is covered by the foreskin (or prepuce), but eight out of ten boys in the United States have this removed a few days after birth.

The reason for this practice was originally religious, and it is still customary for Jews and Muslims. Many doctors believe that there are hygienic advantages in circumcision, but the practice is declining. Some people suppose that circumcision affects the sensitivity of the penis or the boy's ability to control ejaculation, but this is not true.

The two testicles (or testes) which hang below the penis in a sack of loose skin called the scrotum are the glands which produce the male reproductive cells, the sperm (or spermatozoa). They also provide some of the sex hormones which help to bring about the secondary male characteristics at puberty, such as pubic and other body hair, deepening of the voice, and sexual response such as erection.

Once puberty is reached (usually between thirteen and sixteen years of age for boys) millions of sperm 1/500th

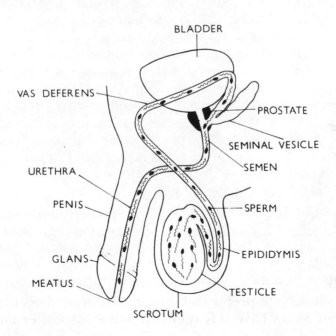

of an inch in length are continually manufactured in the testicles and stored in a coiled tube (the epididymis, at the back of the scrotum. Sperm production is only possible at a temperature somewhat lower than that of the body, and the scrotum adjusts itself so that in warm weather the testicles hang lower, and in colder conditions they are drawn up closer to the body. Normally one testicle hangs slightly lower than the other. Occasionally at birth one or both fail to descend, and if *both* remain within the body no live sperm will be produced and the boy will be sterile (i.e., unable to be a father). This condition can usually be corrected by a doctor.

In erection the penis becomes considerably larger and harder, as a result of increased blood flowing into the spongy tissue. It then points upward and outward from the body and often curves slightly. Erection occurs as a result of physical stimulation in masturbation, petting, or intercourse. But it often happens directly as a result of seeing or just thinking about some sexual object such as a nude picture or a girl you particularly like. Or it may come for a variety of other reasons, some of them entirely nonsexual, such as a full bladder, wearing tight pants, or during an exam or study period. Some boys are worried if they have erections frequently, but this is entirely normal. If there is a physical cause, such as a full bladder, the penis will return to normal as soon as this is removed. If the cause is mental or emotional and erection is awkward the only thing to do is concentrate the mind on something entirely nonsexual. In any case nobody should be troubled by it, and you can't control the penis simply by making up your mind you won't have an erection. Every boy has the same experience, and girls know enough about boys today not to be embarrassed if they happen to notice. There is more cause for concern if a boy by his mid-teens does not have erections at any time. This is very uncommon, and can usually be corrected, but impotence, as the condition is called, often has complex emotional causes which need professional treatment by a psychiatrist. It can also be due to physical disorders, such as diabetes, which can be medically corrected.

Many boys are even more worried about the size of their penis, and with equally little reason. The *adult* penis varies in length when flaccid from two and a half to four inches and when erect from three and a half to eight inches, the average being between five and seven inches. The size of a growing boy's penis varies greatly. As with other parts of the body the penis may develop early in some cases and late in others. It may reach adult size in adolescence or it may grow later. In any case there is no connection between the general size of a boy's body and the size of his penis: it may be much smaller or much larger in proportion to his other organs. Nor is there any direct relation between the size of the penis when soft and when erect, though in the erect state differences in size between individuals tend to be reduced. Finally, the size of the penis does not affect a man's capacity to reach erection or ejaculate, his enjoyment of orgasm, or his ability to give sexual satisfaction to a girl.

Orgasm is the intensely pleasurable climax to sexual arousal, in which increasing muscular and nervous tension, affecting the breathing and heartbeat as well as the genitals, is suddenly released in violent physical spasms. It is followed by a sense of satisfaction and loss of erection, but young men can usually have more than one orgasm after renewed stimulation. In the healthy adolescent or adult it is the muscular rhythms of orgasm that provide the pressure for ejaculation. During ejaculation several hundred million sperm pass along a duct inside the body (the vas deferens), become mixed with a sticky whitish fluid called semen, and spurt out through the urethra and the meatus. The urethra serves also as the channel for passing urine, but when the penis is erect and prepared for ejaculation valves cut off the tube leading to the bladder, so that water cannot be passed.

Orgasm can be experienced long before ejaculation is possible, and the first ejaculation of semen takes place six months to a year before the first sperm are produced. A man may be able to have orgasm and ejaculate even though he may be infertile (incapable of reproduction because his testicles are not producing live sperm). This condition, unlike impotence, is purely physical in origin, but it can often be corrected medically.

Many boys first experience ejaculation during nocturnal emissions or wet dreams. Those who have not been told in advance about this may be worried or frightened, but it is a perfectly normal indication that the sexual powers of puberty are starting to work. At least seven boys out of every ten have wet dreams in their teens. Whether the causes are psychological or physical is not known for certain, but it is usually accompanied by fantasies of some sexual type. Emissions may occur several times a week, twice a month, or less frequently. On waking there may be a feeling of fatigue or a mild ache in the genitals, but these effects soon pass. Since wet dreams are entirely beyond our control and have no harmful consequences, they should be accepted without anxiety or guilt of any kind. They do not involve any loss of sexual power and they are not caused or increased by masturbation. If anything, those who masturbate are less likely to have wet dreams. There is nothing comparable in the girl's experience, and nocturnal emissions in no way correspond to ovulation or menstruation.

The Female Sex Organs

The girl's genitals are more internally situated than those of the boy. The external covering, or vulva, between the legs, consists of two folds of skin and tissue called the

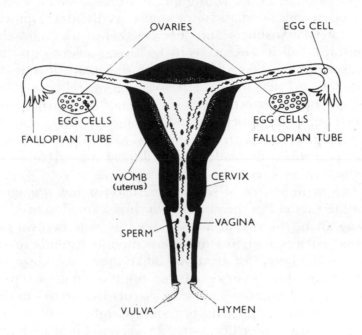

labia majora and the labia minora. Within these are three
quite distinct organs: the clitoris (nearest the front of the
body), the urethra through which urine from the bladder
passes, and the vagina. The vagina is the major female
sex organ, in which intercourse takes place, and through
which a baby is born. It is normally rather like an unin-
flated balloon about six inches in length from the outer
opening of the vulva to the cervix at the entrance to the
womb or uterus. It is capable of expanding to many times
the original size—sufficiently to allow a baby's head to
emerge at birth.

The entrance to the vagina is usually covered by a thin
membrane called the hymen, and traditionally the presence of an unbroken hymen has been regarded as evidence of virginity in a woman. Some authorities believe
that the hymen serves the purpose of decreasing early

sexual arousal in the young girl and thus allows a longer
period in childhood and adolescence for the development
of maternal instincts and less physically oriented relationships. But its absence is by no means a sure sign that
intercourse has taken place. In the first place it must be
remembered that the hymen does not entirely cover the
vaginal opening, otherwise the normal menstrual flow
which starts at puberty could not escape. In some instances girls are born without any hymen. In others it
may be broken or made pliable during masturbation or
petting, or as a result of using tampons.

The main source of sexual pleasure for the woman is
not the vagina but the clitoris, which is a small mound of
tissue about the size of a pea. Like the male penis it becomes enlarged when stimulated, though it tends to re-
tract at the height of arousal. Unlike the penis, however,
the clitoris plays no essential role in intercourse or reproduction, and nothing similar to ejaculation occurs in the
female. However, female orgasm, brought about by the
stimulation of the clitoral area in masturbation or intercourse, can be as intensely satisfying as in the male, and
may be more quickly reached, sustained for longer, and
more easily repeated.

The female sex cell, egg, or ovum (plural: ova) is much
larger than the male sperm, but still only a quarter the
size of the period at the end of this sentence. At birth the
female child has several hundred thousand ova in the two
ovaries which are located on either side of the uterus in
the middle of the pelvis. By puberty the number is reduced to about 10,000 in each ovary; but since no woman
uses more than four or five hundred in her reproductive
life the supply is always sufficient. Between the ages of
twelve and fifteen the ovaries begin to release mature
ova, normally one each month from each ovary in turn.
The egg travels down a duct (the Fallopian tube) and

then (unless it is fertilized by a male sperm) into the pear-shaped uterus where it disintegrates.

The sex hormone in the ovary anticipates the possibility of fertilization every month by building up in the womb additional tissue and blood which can provide the necessary conditions for the growth of a baby. Actually this process may begin a year or more before ovulation (the release of a mature ovum), so that menstruation does not necessarily indicate that a girl is immediately capable of becoming pregnant. If fertilization does not take place, the additional layer of tissue and blood (normally about three tablespoonfuls, but sometimes as little as two or as much as ten) is discharged through the vagina.

Three common misunderstandings about menstruation need to be firmly corrected. First, although the process takes on the average three to five days, there is nothing abnormal or significant if it lasts up to seven days. Longer periods should be discussed with a doctor, and if necessary medical treatment can correct the problem. Second, although the word *menstruation* is derived from the Latin word for month, clockwork regularity is far less common than many books suggest. Particularly during the first years of menstruation, periods are often late or early, or in some cases one may be missed entirely without any apparent cause. Finally, cramps, headaches, emotional tension, and other temporary disturbances are far from uncommon, especially during adolescence. Severe pain should be reported to a doctor for treatment, but minor discomfort should give no cause for anxiety.

Intercourse and Fertilization

During intercourse the erect penis is inserted into the vagina, and thrust up and down until the male reaches orgasm and his semen and sperm are ejaculated vigorously into the vagina. The most common (though by no means the only satisfactory) arrangement is for the female to lie on her back, legs apart, and for the male to lie above her, face to face.

If the hymen has not been previously ruptured or made pliable there will be a little bleeding. In a few instances the hymen is unusually tough and penetration is impossible. In such cases a minor surgical operation has to be performed by a doctor. Usually the process of petting, which precedes intercourse and which prepares the male by arousing him to erection, is sufficient to produce a natural lubrication of the vagina; but in some cases the use of cold cream or a similar substance is necessary.

Once ejaculation has taken place (and past a certain point the mechanism is beyond the boy's control) several hundred million sperm are forced out of the penis and into the vagina. Many of these make their way into the womb and then into the Fallopian tubes. While it is, of course, impossible to become pregnant through kissing or petting, it is possible even if intercourse has been interrupted or incomplete. If the boy withdraws before he has his orgasm some sperm may escape during the earlier stages of penetration. Even if the girl's hymen is intact, sperm may enter the vagina if they are deposited at the entrance.

Within a few hours of ejaculation many thousand sperm propelled by the rapid whipping of their tails reach the Fallopian tubes. If they here encounter a live ovum (within twenty-four to thirty-six hours of discharge from the ovary), one sperm penetrates the female cell and its nucleus unites with that of the ovum to bring about the conception of a new unit of life. This fertilized egg begins very soon to divide into new cells and starts the slow journey down the Fallopian tube into the womb. About a week later the zygote (as it is technically called to this point) attaches itself to the lining of the womb from which it receives the resources necessary for continued growth. Incoming nourishment and outgoing waste pass between the mother and the embryo through the umbilical cord attached at the navel.

At one month old the embryo is pea-sized. By three months the fetus (as it is now called) is about three inches long and surrounded by a fluid-filled sac (the amniotic sac) which helps to protect it. The main body features can now be identified. By the end of five months the heartbeat can be heard with proper instruments and the mother may feel the fetus move. Birth normally takes place through the vagina nine months after conception.

During pregnancy ovulation ceases, and the absence of normal menstruation is usually the first indication that conception has taken place. Missing a period is not, however, proof that a girl is pregnant. Deep emotional disturbance (including fear of an unwanted pregnancy) can cause a period to be delayed or missed. A simple urine test in a doctor's office or clinic can determine whether a girl is pregnant two weeks after her first missed period. A more complicated (and more expensive) blood test can tell within a few days after intercourse whether fertilization has taken place.

2 · Discovering Sex

I have already emphasized that sex is not something that starts at a particular age, or something we can decide to have or not to have. On the other hand there is a particular time when we become aware of our sexual urges, when our bodies reach a stage of development at which we are capable of reproduction. At this time, called puberty, from the Latin word for *groin*, we discover sex as a physical reality. This chapter is about that exciting but sometimes disturbing experience.

One difficulty with puberty is that nothing happens just the same for any two people. The signs of physical sexual maturity come at different times for each sex and at different times for individual members of each sex. Bodies which seem to have made pretty even growth up to now suddenly go berserk and can't be counted on at all; the order and speed at which different organs mature is entirely unpredictable. Girls generally show the first signs of puberty a couple of years before boys—sometimes as early as nine or ten. But there's nothing wrong if menstruation doesn't begin until sixteen or seventeen. Between ages eleven and thirteen, girls are usually taller than boys of their own age, and this is one reason why they prefer to date rather older boys (another is that girls are usually more mature socially and intellectually at this stage). Boys may have their first wet dreams as early as ten or eleven, or they may not ejaculate until the late teens. A girl may find that her breasts enlarge much earlier or much later than her friends'—or that one develops before the other; it's no more unusual than the fact that some people grow to full height by sixteen while others spurt up years later. A boy often worries because his penis seems much larger or smaller than others' in his class; but it's no more peculiar than the way one's arms or feet seem out of proportion to everything for a while.

When you are at this stage of being least sure of yourself physically, everything is further complicated by the upsurge of strong sexual drives involving the whole personality. And while the first conscious awareness of sex (which, as we have noted, is actually present from the beginning of our existence) gives a wonderful new zest to life, it can lead to anxiety and confusion because of ignorance or false fears.

Puberty Problems of the Boy

Boys are much more conscious of the demands of sex at puberty, and the solution of sexual needs is much more urgent for them than it is for girls. The first sign that something new is stirring within is often a nocturnal emission or wet dream. Soon after this (or, sometimes, before) a boy discovers that he can obtain new pleasure and eventually orgasm through masturbation—the stimulation of the penis with the hands. Often it first serves as a means of inducing sleep at night, then as a relief from the growing internal tensions of sexual desire. Although many boys imagine they are the only ones to engage in this activity it is in fact practiced at some time by ninety-five out of every hundred males in the population, and probably by eight out of ten before the age of fourteen.

Indeed it is now recognized that masturbation, including orgasm, is common in very young children, although at that age, and in the early teens before semen is produced, there is no ejaculation. For centuries, due to mistaken ideas about sexuality, masturbation has been regarded as something to be ashamed of in our society—"self-abuse," to use one popular word for it. Even today many parents react emotionally when a young boy handles his genitals, and this implants in him an unconscious sense of guilt which affects him when the pleasure of masturbation is discovered at puberty. Many adolescents with such ingrained fears go through agonies of worry and self-condemnation because when they find masturbation enjoyable, they think themselves degenerate.

It cannot be emphasized strongly enough that *medical and psychological authorities regard these fears as entirely without foundation.* Most of them would say that, far from being self-abuse, masturbation is a normal (though not essential) stage of self-discovery and self-growth, a natural response to the upsurge of sexual powers in the human body. It is an extension of the process by which in earlier childhood you discovered the limits of your body by exploring toes and hands and ears. It is the means whereby most boys discover the pleasure of sex, and move forward in the crucial process of establishing their identity as male human beings. At the same time it provides a safety-valve for the release of sexual tensions which, particularly in our advanced society, cannot be satisfied immediately with intercourse. If every time a boy needed sexual relief he had to find some girl to sleep with (willingly or otherwise), there would be a great deal more tragedy and sorrow than there is now. Masturbation should be accepted as an inseparable part of adolescent self-exploration and experimentation, a phase in which a boy is preparing for relationships with the other sex.

Does Masturbation Cause Physical Damage?

Boys often worry that they get pimples or acne as the result of masturbation, or that they can rupture themselves or permanently reduce their physical resources by frequent masturbation. There is absolutely no basis in fact for any of these fears.* The idea that all sorts of bodily ailments result from masturbation seems to have been invented, or at least made popular, by an anonymous quack who wanted to sell a patent medicine to cure the diseases that he claimed resulted from self-indulgence. "If we turn our eyes on licentious Masturbators," he wrote, "we shall find them with meagre Jaws and pale Looks, with feeble Hams and legs without Calves, their generative faculties weakened if not destroyed in the Prime of their Years; a Jest to others and a Torment to themselves." His theory was taken up by more respected medical authorities, who found in it a new weapon to support traditional religious objections. In 1879 Dr. J. H. Kellogg, the inventor of cornflakes, attributed lassitude, sleeplessness, bashfulness, unnatural boldness, mock piety, confusion of ideas, round shoulders, weak backs, paralysis, the use of tobacco, moist hands, palpitation of the heart, hysteria, epilepsy, bed-wetting, impotence, dyspepsia, cancer, insanity, and suicide to masturbation. Not until the 1940s did the medical profession finally abandon these totally unfounded ideas.

Hardly any doctor today will say that masturbation is physically damaging, but some imply that it is harmful "in excess." However, this information is more likely to result in greater anxiety than less, for a boy is seldom told what constitutes "excess." He is left to worry endlessly about whether he has done it too much and caused himself per-

---

*Teenage acne is caused by the operation of certain oil glands during adolescence and has no sexual meaning at all.

manent damage. But in fact it is impossible to masturbate so much as to injure the body. There is a point at which the nervous responses which lead to orgasm become exhausted, and this is well before any harm can be done to the system. When that point comes depends upon the individual, and it varies greatly. Some boys in early adolescence masturbate several times in a day, others only infrequently, a few never. The physical effects are no more serious or permanent than eating a heavy meal or playing a tough game of football. There is a temporary loss of energy and reduction of tension, but the body makes up the deficiency in a few hours. This means that the boy who needs to be fully fit for a track meet or alert for an exam will usually be sensible not to masturbate immediately before. But in some cases the reduction of tension may be helpful, and it's certainly wiser to enjoy a sound night's sleep before some crucial event than to spend a restless night trying to fight off a need for sexual release.

Does Masturbation Cause Sexual Damage?

Some early psychoanalysts thought that masturbation could reduce sexual powers, but this is now known to be untrue. The sperm which are necessary for conception are continually being produced by the testicles: there is no limited store to be exhausted by any amount of sexual activity. On the whole the evidence suggests that those who begin sexual activity early continue it longest and engage in it most vigorously. Masturbation cannot make you infertile (or, for that matter, make you fertile if you are not). It may conceivably lead to some minor enlargement of the penis if frequently practiced; but the size of the male organ is irrelevant to sexual satisfaction or performance in intercourse later on. The idea that people who have masturbated find it difficult to enjoy intercourse is unfounded. Sometimes men who have difficul-

ties in marriage *suspect* that their earlier habits of masturbation are to blame; but the causes are usually found to
lie in complicated psychological problems unrelated to
the physical act of masturbation.

The plain fact is that every individual has a different
sexual level of need and energy, and there's not much
point in envying those with more powerful urges or those
with weaker ones. Generally good health and sound
habits of eating, sleeping, and exercise are the best way to
ensure a satisfying sexual life. You can exercise some control over the *type* of sexual activity you engage in, but the
basic urge to sexual expression is something you are born
with and have to live with. Particularly the extent to
which your system seems to demand relief in masturbation should be accepted without anxiety or fear.

Does Masturbation Cause Mental or Psychological Damage?

Once again the answer is firmly in the negative, although
for centuries fear of insanity was used as a threat to dis-
courage masturbation, and such warnings are not unknown today. The reason is probably that, before the development of modern methods of treatment, the insane
were observed to masturbate publicly. Now we know that
public masturbation by adults is a symptom of mental disorder; it is in no sense a cause of it. Among adolescents
masturbation may sometimes be used as a substitute for
facing up to personal problems, fears of inadequacy,
pressures at school, or conflicts with one's parents. It is
not the cause of these difficulties, but it may be an excuse
for avoiding a realistic and honest solution of them. In
such a case professional help is advisable and can usually
lead to a resolution of the problem.

Three out of every four boys engage in some kind of
fantasy during masturbation. That is, the boy thinks

about some girl he knows—or sometimes about an older woman—and imagines himself petting or having intercourse with her. Often he feels especially guilty or disgusted at himself for this and wonders whether it indicates some perversion. Most psychiatrists, on the contrary, think fantasy a healthy sign. If masturbatory fantasies are exclusively concentrated on one's own sex or involve ideas of inflicting pain on people, they may again be symptoms (not causes) of underlying troubles. But it can be argued that masturbation that is a purely physical and mechanical pleasure, concentrating attention on the boy's own genitals, is more self-centered and infantile than masturbation which includes hopes and dreams of eventual relations with another person. At the same time it is important that the fantasy be recognized for what it is and that the boy be able to distinguish it from reality.

Does Masturbation Cause Spiritual Damage?

The religious objection to masturbation was for centuries based on the Old Testament story of Onan (Genesis 38) who, according to the story, "spilled his seed upon the ground" and was punished by God for doing so. It is now widely recognized that Onan's "sin" was not masturbation but a failure to fulfill the custom of the day by having intercourse with the widow of his dead brother so that she could have a child. Many religious authorities now recognize that masturbation in itself is spiritually harmless. Even Catholic teaching, which has been most condemnatory, is now being modified in the light of modern knowledge. Traditional religious fears have lost much of their power because we now know that the great emphasis by preachers and priests on the supposed physical or mental disasters resulting from masturbation is nonsense.

Each individual will have to make up his or her own mind, in the light of religious convictions and accurate information, whether masturbation is spiritually harmful or not. But two things can be said which may help. First, people with strong religious convictions are able to restrain the impulse to masturbation more successfully than others, though the number of males who avoid it altogether is small. Second, anyone who feels it is sinful to masturbate will only cause himself unnecessary anxiety and guilt if he ignores what his conscience tells him is right. In other words, if you really feel it *is* wrong to masturbate you should try to control it. The avoidance of sexually stimulating sights or situations, disciplined concentration of the mind on other things, vigorous physical activity and spiritual exercises may help. But if you believe masturbation is sinful and want to fight it, don't make the problem larger than necessary by imagining that you are alone in what has been called "the solitary vice." Almost every boy or man you know has engaged in the practice at some time or other.

Personally it seems to me that if we accepted masturbation (as many societies do) as a natural phenomenon of puberty, no more sinful than menstruation, most of the anxiety and fear it generates would never arise. As it is, by concentrating a great deal of moral and religious effort on avoiding something that is part of healthy sexual development, many teenagers divert their spiritual resources from more important and manageable problems. In my opinion, religious teachers would do better to tell their members that masturbation is to be welcomed as God's provision of a temporary substitute for the full joys of sexual intercourse, so that no religious guilt should accompany it at all. Even some Catholic authorities are now beginning to accept this position.

At the same time it seems probable that masturbation will always leave feelings of dissatisfaction and disappointment. The purely physical experience of orgasm may be overwhelming for someone quite unprepared for it: he may fear that something disastrous (though also enjoyable) has gone wrong with his body. If he's ill-informed he may fear that his sexual powers have been dissipated, and this emotional shock may be difficult to obliterate. Again, masturbation is often the first occasion on which the adolescent rejects what he knows to be parental wishes and finds the result pleasant instead of painful. Despite the necessity of beginning to live his own life, there is an unavoidable hurt in the breaking of childhood relationships to his parents.

It is important to move on eventually from masturbation, which is solitary, to sexual experience, which is interpersonal. If there were no feeling of dissatisfaction about masturbation, some boys might not progress beyond private self-satisfaction to the greater possibilities of interpersonal love. They might remain fixated at the level of self-love instead of graduating into relations with other people. So, while accepting masturbation as a stage of growth, it should be recognized as a relatively immature level of sexual progress.

Puberty Problems of the Girl

The outward signs of puberty often come upon the girl more unexpectedly than upon the boy, and when they do arrive they can be more terrifying if she is not prepared. She should be prepared by the first budding of her breasts and the appearance of pubic hair in the genital area, but if she has been given no advance information about menstruation it can be embarrassing and frightening. A girl who is not forewarned may think she has damaged herself through masturbation or petting, or fear that she has cancer or is giving birth to a baby. It's important to recognize that menstruation is a natural, healthy function of the body and nothing to fear or be ashamed of. The idea that girls are "cursed" by it is a hangover from primitive superstition. To think of it as a sign of feminine "weakness" is pure male delusion, for very few men could accept the inconvenience and occasional discomfort of the monthly period without perpetual complaining. As one anthropologist put it, the only superior physical strength men have is the capacity to kill a cow with one blow—in every other respect women are potentially stronger, putting up with more hardship, adjusting better to difficult conditions, surviving worse illnesses, and living longer than men.

But even with the best preparation and knowledge menstruation is a nuisance for many girls, and human relationships would be much happier if boys were aware of the nature of the experience their mothers and sisters and girl friends go through. During menstruation some stomach cramps, slight headache, or backache are by no means uncommon. Not every girl can wear a tampon, and sanitary napkins are sometimes uncomfortable. *Excessive* fatigue is best avoided, although moderate exercise and all other regular activities can be enjoyed. There are emotional effects due to the working of the sex hormones, and these can cause irritability, anxiety, and nervousness. Studies have shown that girls often do less than their best work academically during menstruation. Moreover, periods are quite often irregular and liable to upset the best-planned schedule, especially in the early years. Anxiety over the health of a parent or over a forthcoming test, the excitement of traveling or minor sickness can all delay the process. Despite the fears of some girls, there is actually no way in which a boy can tell if a girl is menstruating; but life would be easier if boys were more responsive to the comment, "I don't feel myself today."

Inevitably the different way that puberty affects the body of the boy or girl affects the way each feels about the experience. The boy is actively and happily engaged in discovering the early signs of manhood in the capacity to achieve erection and ejaculation. The girl is more the passive subject of a change which comes *upon* her and seems to represent a loss and an inconvenience. Ultimately, women are more confident and secure in their sexuality than men, and the biological basis of human life is originally female rather than male. But in early adolescence there is no way in which a girl can objectively confirm her sexuality. The capacity for childbearing, which later on will be a source of deep sexual assurance for many women, is better *not* demonstrated in the teens. But unfortunately many girls find it very difficult to wait until adulthood to gain inner confidence in their personal identity. The result is that they seek, consciously or unconsciously, to prove themselves by motherhood and become pregnant long before they are socially and psychologically (let alone economically) prepared for this responsibility.

Masturbation does not play the same part in the girl's development at puberty as it does for the boy; although a girl can experience orgasm, through stimulation of the clitoris, as readily as a boy. It is estimated that eventually six out of every ten women masturbate. But in the teens the proportion is much smaller—only one out of every four girls has masturbated to orgasm by fifteen, compared with nine out of ten boys. Perhaps because her genitals are more interior and less easily stimulated, the female seems to need sexual relief through orgasm much less at this age than does the male. Whereas a boy's sexuality is concentrated largely on the genitals in puberty, a girl's sexuality is much more diffuse and permeates her whole being. Girls' sexual needs, like those of boys, vary greatly, and while there is nothing unnatural or harmful in teenage masturbation, there is no reason to be worried if one feels no particular interest in or desire for this activity. Whereas males reach the peak of their sexual vigor in the late teens, and most teenage boys want to "go all the way" then, girls are much slower to develop similar physical needs. During the early teens most girls are sexually satisfied by social contacts with boys and the less intimate physical pleasures such as kissing, hugging, and necking.

3 · Becoming a Person

At puberty you become capable of reproduction, but you are obviously not capable of fulfilling parental responsibilities just because you are capable of becoming a father or mother. Boys and girls of twelve or thirteen can produce children, but nobody imagines they are ready to take care of them. Between physical sexual maturity and psychological maturity you have to live through adolescence—the more drawn-out stage in which you develop the personal qualities and attitudes that will mark your adult life.

Of course, it is not a simple matter of making up your mind, according to some ideal picture, what you will be like and then magically acquiring the qualities you want to have. You are already partly formed as a person through the various experiences of childhood, and the instinctive forces of nature cannot be merely ignored or blocked without serious consequences. Nevertheless in adolescence you do have some capacity to affect the formation of your character. Puberty, it has been said, is an act of nature: adolescence is an act of humans. Many people fail to make much use of this opportunity, because of ignorance or laziness; but it is the unique privilege of the human species to have some part in determining the direction of its own development. We are not the prisoners of our past experiences or our past behavior: in the teens surprising new attitudes and personal qualities emerge, and the more you understand what is going on the better you will be able to come through the turmoil of adolescence as a free and mature person.

The Turmoil of Adolescence

The first thing to realize is that turmoil is a normal part of the process of becoming an adult and few, even in the darkest hour, would really want to return to the security and simplicity of childhood. But whereas the growth of the body more or less automatically brings physical maturity, becoming a mature person is far less inevitable and can be delayed or distorted much more easily. Most of the sexual troubles that people suffer from arise from the fact that they have become adults in the legal or biological sense without becoming mature mentally and emotionally. Their bodies are full grown and their sexual drives are vigorous, but their personalities and relationships remain stunted or deformed. They are physical men and women but psychological infants.

Until puberty, close ties with parents and family are a necessary support, enabling the child to develop human qualities, values, and ideals. It is the greatly extended dependency period in human growth that enables us to learn what personal relationships and social responsibilities mean. Other animals become independent much sooner, but they lack man's unique capacity for personhood. Unless and until you become free of childhood bonds and begin to organize your own life around your own chosen ideals, you are not fully human. Any boy or girl who is a mere carbon copy of his or her parents has not become a person. And independence is seldom achieved without some tensions and in many cases violent crisis. However understanding and sensible parents may be, there are always some points about which their expectations and standards will differ from those of their children. Often it is in utterly unimportant things that the conflict first shows itself, such as the length of a boy's hair or the shortness of a girl's skirt. The very fact that it is in such matters of taste (about which little rational argument is possible) that the generations part company shows that it is not so much the issue that is important as the separation—the declaration of independence by the individual boy or girl. Nor does independence necessarily mean a final repudiation of parental standards. Sociological studies indicate that two out of every three people find that their own mature values are very close to those of their parents. But what matters is that they are now their own. They have been challenged and tested and eventually embraced because they seem more adequate and meaningful to the individual concerned, not merely out of fear or respect for parental wishes.

Reaching for Independence

Becoming a person means establishing some coherent self-identity, accepting responsibility for your own actions, knowing what you want to do and be. It doesn't mean that you have succeeded or will succeed in living up 100 percent to what you think right or desirable. It does mean that you are able to make some judgment about your behavior based on your own conscience. It means that you feel guilty or unhappy or unworthy when you act contrary to what *you* believe to be right. A sense of guilt which is due to failure to live according to some standard imposed from without by parents or society can be morbid and destructive of human freedom. But on the other hand, people who lack *any* sense of wrongdoing, technically called psychopaths, are recognized by psychiatrists as less than fully human persons, and they frequently end up as habitual criminals. People vary enormously in the content they give to conscience and in the things for which they feel guilt, but becoming a person involves at least some clarification of values, goals, and ideals to which you are committed.

Sexuality plays a major role in the achievement of personal independence, and the identity established in adolescence is profoundly concerned with knowing what it is to be a man or a woman. The critical point of debate over parental control will often be the hour at which dates are to end or the amount of supervision to be imposed at parties. In every generation the sexual standards of the young appear too liberal to their elders, even though the parents enjoyed greater freedom when they were young than they want to grant their children. Studies have shown that parents become increasingly strict about sexual behavior as their children become teenagers, and it seems that each generation may need this contrast if adolescents are to develop healthy independence. A boy or a girl whose parents are entirely permissive may find it harder to establish sexual standards of his or her own because he has nothing against which to affirm his own different point of view. You need something to rebel against, to flex your moral muscles, and both parents and children would be saved a lot of unnecessary pain if they accepted this give-and-take as part of the normal process of growing up. I'm not saying that adults serve merely as useful sparring partners, for older people do have experience and knowledge teenagers lack, and it is just as foolish to brush it all off as it is to accept their opinions without question.

But deeper issues are involved than the mere question of standards and regulations. Parents and children are bound together by profound unconscious ties which go back to early childhood and cannot be broken without emotional costs. A young boy goes through a stage of attachment to his mother which is sexual (though not genital) in character, and may sometimes be expressed in jealousy of the father. "I want to sleep with mummy" is a common protest in a four- or five-year old, and he vaguely thinks of father as a rival. He learns soon enough (if the parents are themselves sexually mature and understanding) that this is not possible, and transfers his affection to his father, taking him as the model for his *future* sexual role. A girl between four and six develops a passionate attachment to her father, and tries to take her mother's place. Once again, provided the parents neither indulge the child's fantasies nor treat them as morally wrong and react with disgust or coldness, the girl learns that she is not yet ready to assume the female sexual role and identifies herself for the time being with her mother as her ideal. But at puberty both the original attraction to the parent of the other sex and the temporary identification with the parent of the same sex have to be faced again and finally left behind if mature sexuality is to be achieved. It has been well said that "Falling out of love with parents is the first step toward falling in love with a mate."

And this can be very difficult and painful, leading to moodiness, depression, and insecurity. For a girl finally to abandon her childhood relation to her father and begin to learn to love a man of her own age, while at the same time accepting for herself the adult role of womanhood previously filled in the family by her mother, rouses hidden anxieties. If a father persists in treating his daughter as *his* little girl at the age of seventeen, her capacity for adult sexual relationships with a man may be impaired. Equally, the boy who remains in a childhood relation to his mother may never break away from her apron strings and develop sexual relations with a girl. Some mothers are so critical of a son's date—perhaps because they feel their own bond to him is threatened—that it may be difficult for the boy to establish a continuing relationship with a girl. Usually the dynamics of sexual growth and the good sense of parents bring about a healthy solution: but it is as well to realize that the petty conflicts and emotional tangles that upset adolescent relations with mother or father are the surface indications of an inner struggle for sexual and personal freedom. It may be only when an appropriate sexual partner has been found that a mature relationship of mutual love and respect with the parent can be re-established. We can't avoid or fully understand these hidden conflicts, but we may save ourselves a lot of pain if we recognize their existence and remember that they are usually temporary.

The Influence of Peers

In our society the peer group—the adolescent world, the gang, the group of close friends—plays a major part in the process of achieving personal independence. Most teenagers are not ready to break away immediately from the family circle and assert their individuality on their own; they need the support and strength that others in the same situation as themselves can offer. In American life the importance of the peer group is greater than in almost any culture in the world. In more primitive societies the task of preparing a boy or girl for adult life was largely supervised by adults, even when great sexual freedom was officially permitted within the adolescent group itself. In other parts of the world today there is much more continuing contact between a teenager and his parents or other adults in social affairs than in America. The availability of automobiles and the financial prosperity which allows teenagers to choose their own clothes and entertainment, or among the less affluent the breakdown of family life which forces young people out of crowded tenements into street gangs, tend to establish self-contained units in which standards of behavior are developed in isolation from the "tuned-out" world of the over-thirties. There are some advantages in this, insofar as the danger of remaining too closely tied to one's parents is reduced. But it may threaten the development of the individual's unique personal potential. It is just as easy to become a mere conformist to the values and habits of a particular teenage group as it is to remain a conformist to parental standards. You are not really a free person so long as you are meekly following the dictates of your particular crowd, any more than you are when you meekly follow the rules laid down by your parents.

Because sexual issues are so central to the establishment of self-identity and independence, it is particularly difficult not to go along with the group when it acts in revolt against adult rules. Where there are limits on sexual behavior set up by authority, a teenager who exercises restraint may seem a traitor to his peers. But it is important to remember that those with the most highly developed interest in sexual experimentation usually set the pace. This may not be because they have the greatest sexual powers, but perhaps because they need the greatest reassurance and want the support of being *thought* advanced. Studies have shown that the tendency of any teenage group is to stimulate and enforce aggressive behavior, even among those who have little stomach for it individually. So a truly free person will keep in mind the great differences in sexual development during adolescence and make his or her own pace. It may mean some teasing and occasional loneliness; but the boy or girl whose sexual development is strong and mature will be able to resist the temptation to make a big "score" or join a group that goes in for casual, impersonal sex. However difficult it may be, if you want to develop your own personality to the full you won't automatically conform to the principle of "the sooner the better, the bigger the better, the faster the better."

Is Restraint Dangerous?

Becoming a person means more than breaking away from childhood restraints and achieving independent identity; it means learning to exercise some control over your natural instincts so that you are free to attain whatever ideals and goals you feel to be of first importance. The boy or girl who wants to be an actor or astronaut or teacher or doctor or millionaire has to make decisions about the use of time and energy in order to acquire the necessary skills. Anyone who wants to achieve sexual maturity and to enjoy the full human satisfactions of sex has to learn to restrain or direct the sexual urge.

But wait a minute, someone says. Isn't it harmful to repress your sexual desires? Isn't it important to fulfill your bodily needs as soon as they become insistent, whether you are thirteen or fifteen or seventeen? Doesn't abstinence from sex lead to all sorts of distorted guilt feelings that foul up your personality? The answer is that everything depends on the *reasons* for restraint, and the kind of control you are talking about. The idea that abstinence impairs one's capacities for subsequent sexual performance is a teenage myth without any scientific basis. If you avoid all sexual activity because of prohibitions imposed by other people, or because you are unable to accept the fact that sex is good in itself, or because you can't bring yourself to have any dealings with the other sex, then certainly sexual abstinence may be bad. Even then, the underlying confusion in your thinking and feeling has to be cleared up rather than the symptom. Just engaging in sex without any change of attitude will not solve the problem. But if you deliberately choose to limit your sexual activity because you have other goals in mind, then restraint may be a sign of maturity and strength. There are surely things any human being ought to feel guilty about. If you are incapable of realizing the pain we can cause other people and the damage we do to our own selves by purely selfish sexual acts, you aren't truly a person. There is nothing psychologically abnormal or distorted in feeling shame when you fail to treat another person as a human being and force your attentions on them when they don't respond. Nobody would think it healthy for a man to rape a girl just because he had an overwhelming urge to engage in intercourse. Some self-control in the interests of other people consistent with your own personal standards is obviously essential. So the girl who chooses to remain a virgin because she wants to share intercourse only with the man she marries, and the boy who restrains himself from heavy petting out of concern of his date's feelings are not harming themselves. They are acting as responsible persons, not as moral infants or psychopaths.

Differences in Sexual Needs

It is sometimes said that sex is a need like hunger which must be satisfied. The ads for one movie showed a man apparently assaulting a girl, with the statement "There are some hungers no man can resist." It is true that our sexual needs often have the same kind of insistence and urgency about them that our need for food has. But this does not mean that everybody has the same need for sexual satisfaction or that this need has to be met in one particular way or at one particular time. In the first place, although everyone needs a certain minimum amount of sustenance to keep alive, and needs to eat and drink with some regularity, our requirements for survival differ greatly; the kinds of foods we depend on vary according to where we live, our age, and other factors. We can to a considerable extent control our hunger (or at least we can control the extent to which we satisfy it) without harm to ourselves, as people on diets have to learn. So even if sexual need is as universal as hunger, there's no reason why you should assume that it is beyond any kind of control. Indeed most of us would regard somebody who felt compelled to satisfy his sexual urge immediately that it arose, regardless of circumstances or other concerns, as a pretty weak character—just as we would think a person very stupid who always ate whatever took his fancy at the risk of becoming grossly fat.

Whether it is possible for some people to abstain entirely from sexual activity without harm is an open question. There are some whose sexual drives are so weak, or whose dedication to an ideal of self-denial is so strong (particularly, many priests and nuns), that they are apparently able to live without ever enjoying conscious sexual pleasure. Some would say that their sexual drives are not so much eliminated as redirected or "sublimated" into other forms of self-realization. It certainly seems ridiculous to suggest that all celibates are lacking in sexual identity, or that they are all living impoverished or dishonest lives.

Directing Sexual Drives

The great majority of men and women, however, certainly need some sexual relief, and teenagers (particularly boys) need it quite frequently. For many teenagers the attempt to control all the sexual demands of the body is as impossible as it would be to go without food. But the question is *how* that desire is to be satisfied. Just as you can choose different foods to meet your need of sustenance, so you have choices about the way you satisfy your sexual needs. It is here that character and ideals become relevant. "It is not sexual behavior that determines character," said the psychiatrist Erich Fromm, "but character that determines sexual behavior." You are free to decide whether you will gratify your sexual hunger through masturbation, through petting, or through intercourse. Which of these you use will depend upon the personal values you have established. If you put pleasure or sexual success or your reputation in the peer group first, you may act one way. If your conscience places a high importance on concern for other people or tells you that some kinds of sexual pleasure are only appropriate after marriage, you will behave differently.

The basic sexual urge in man is the direct extension of the reproductive urge in the animal world, without which evolution and life would have petered out millions of years ago. If men did not have an inborn instinct to initiate sexual activity leading to intercourse and conception, and women an equally natural readiness to accept their advances, the race would be defunct. But to argue from this, as some do, that for human beings to exercise conscious direction of their sexual drives according to moral standards and higher values is "unnatural" is absurd. The basic physical sex act is shared by man with the animal world; but its significance and meaning has been enlarged and greatly complicated by the development of human personality.

What most clearly distinguishes human sexuality is the fact that the female is no longer a mere convenience for male satisfaction or a bearer of offspring. Women have a unique capacity for sexual pleasure and men make a conscious commitment to those with whom they mate, traits unknown in the animal world. To talk about treating sex as an animal instinct alone is to imply that women should be treated as inferior creatures to serve men's pleasure, and bear their children. Of course, there are people (usually men) who think and act as if that's all sex is; but most people find such an attitude unsatisfying. Moreover, the history of human biological and sociological development suggests that such a view of sex is a step backward on the evolutionary ladder. In the rest of the animal world, for example, the female is sexually receptive only for a very brief period when she is ovulating and liable to become pregnant, whereas among humans women may be interested in sexual contact at any time, and they are often most responsive just before or after menstruation when conception is *least* likely. It appears that subhuman females probably do not experience orgasm: there it is a male prerogative. Only among humans does the female enjoy sex fully. In other primates, except to some extent the chimpanzees, sex is inseparable from dominance and aggression. Once again, we find this attitude to sex among men; but it is distinctively human to regard intercourse as a union of equals rather than the conquest of the inferior by the superior. Finally, although "pair formation" is not unique to humans, it is not known among other primates, and the sexual union of marriage has a permanence and a mutuality of a special kind. The degree to which males in the human species share in the nurturing role of the family, and to some extent depend on the female for their own survival, has no parallel in other species.

Responsibility for Each Other

What this all adds up to is the fact that human life has a dimension of personal relationship, respect, love, commitment, which is absent from the rest of the animal world. Psychiatrists emphasize that without sound relationships to others we cannot become mature persons. You are not an isolated, self-contained unit. You only grow psychologically and emotionally if your personal relations with others are sound and constructive. Throughout adolescence you are learning to relate to people as people, to treat them as your equals, and to develop your individual identity in the context of open relationships.

This means that becoming a person in the fullest sense of the word is inconsistent with an impersonal use of sex. Boys or girls who trick or lie or coerce or exploit people sexually are demonstrating that they have not yet become persons. They are not only wronging the other person by treating him or her as a mere thing, they are reducing their own humanity to the level of beasts.

We hear a lot about rape these days. You can hardly watch television for a day or go to the movies for a month without some reference to it. Most people in our society react with abhorrence to the idea of forcing another person to engage in sex. Despite the accusation of some women, it is probably not true that all men are rapists deep down—through as a male I have to admit that my opinion is possibly a cover-up. But it is certainly true that many women and many teenage girls are victims of "soft rape" or "civilized rape"—of situations in which they are, in effect, placed under such psychological pressure that it is difficult for them to resist the male's advances. Boys (and occasionally girls) who force someone against her (or his) better judgment to engage in intercourse, even if no overt physical force is used, are surely falling below the level of human personhood.

Exactly when a sexual relationship is truly personal or when it is superficial or immature we still have to consider, and that is a much more difficult question to answer. The attainment of a consistent, unified personality is the goal toward which adolescence points, and few reach adulthood without mistakes they regret and experiences that are painful. What matters most is to have some idea of where you want to go, and to realize how profoundly your sexual values and actions will affect your personal maturity.

4 · Discovering the Other Sex

Unfortunately you don't have the opportunity to establish your own independent identity and values *before* getting involved in relations with the other sex. Adolescence is complicated by the fact that you have to work out what kind of person you are, and how you relate to the other sex, while you are still in the process of finding out what they are like. Indeed you learn about your own sexuality—what it means to be a boy or a girl—through encountering members of the other sex in all their difference. You learn what it is to be a human being, male or female, through all sorts of interaction with boys *and* girls, girls *and* boys.

Your first meetings with the other sex (outside your own family) are likely to be in social activities, or at school, where at first you are not aware of particular individuals at all. But before long your interest is focused on a select few who attract you especially. At first there may be little direct physical contact, but the relationship is sexual already—and the better for being so. The different ways in which members of the other sex respond to social situations, interpret history, enjoy literature, or play games can help you grow as a person. When you begin to enjoy physical sexual pleasure from the feel or touch of

41

another body, you are developing a perfectly natural range of human experience. When a particular boy or girl responds to your attentions, it is entirely right that this special relationship should be expressed in greater physical intimacy. But discovering the other sex—and discovering what it is to be human—is not as simple as people often imagine.

Although girls normally become sexually mature (in the sense of being capable of parenthood) before boys, it is generally boys who first want physical contact with girls, soon after they reach puberty. As we have seen, masturbation is frequently accompanied by fantasies of petting or intercourse, and provides a preparation for the next stage of sexual maturation. It's important to remember that individuals vary greatly in the age at which they reach puberty, and an adolescent boy may find that while all his friends have begun to date he still lacks any enthusiasm for girls who seem to be silly, awkward, giggly things. Another boy may be interested but because of shyness may take longer to build up courage to ask a girl for a date. Some are too easily discouraged if their first attempts are rebuffed, forgetting that we have to learn to accept disappointments, and that any girl has the right to turn a boy down if she wants. But each has to develop at his own speed, and there's nothing to worry about if it takes longer than you would like to develop contacts with the other sex and the social graces to make them enjoyable. It would certainly help if girls remembered that boys are often anxious and inwardly unsure of themselves when they begin dating, despite the air of bravado they may put on.

The Boy's Sexual Urge

Once a boy has got past the initial embarrassment, however, he is likely to want to progress quite rapidly to physical intimacy. Boys are easily aroused sexually by the way a girl walks or by the way she throws her hair back. Merely thinking about a girl's body, or looking at a nude photograph, or hearing a sexual joke may result in erection. Physical contact, even if it's accidental or a formal goodnight kiss, brings into play the first stages of male sexual response. Flirting or holding hands or sitting close together in a car or at the movies with a girl he likes (whether she cares about him or not) starts off a sequence of stimulation that leads naturally to orgasm. He may not realize what is taking place, but his quite healthy instinct is to maintain and if possible increase the pleasurable tension of his body. Once the mechanism leading to ejaculation has been set in motion a real effort may be needed to avoid completing the cycle. His sexual dynamics propel him to increasingly close exploration of the girl's body, so that the progression from kissing to tongue-kissing, then to fondling the girl's breasts, and eventually to petting and genital contact would be unbroken if it were not for cultural and personal restraints. As a matter of fact, a boy *can* interrupt the sequence, though he may find that he has to obtain relief later through masturbation, or has a wet dream that night. But the important thing for him and for the girl to realize is that quite elementary necking triggers off forces of great strength and pleasure which in later life will be the normal prelude to intercourse. Because a girl, as we shall see, may be quite unaroused in the physical, genital sense, there is no reason for her to react with disgust or contempt—or even with pained surprise! A boy who shows signs of sexual excitement when he's given what is intended to be a friendly hug or a companionable hand to hold is not some kind of monster; he's exhibiting the normal male initiative in sexual activity which has made possible the perpetuation of the human race. Because he's a human being and not just an animal, and because he's engaged in the business of becoming a person, a boy is also usually aware that more is involved than the immediate satisfaction of his bodily desires. However dimly and inadequately, he knows that physical intimacy is part of a wider encounter with a person, and that there is more to a girl than her body.

Necking and Petting

Necking and petting can be means of expressing more than mere sensual attraction; they can communicate affection, admiration, appreciation. Even the first, hesitant explorations of a boy and girl together are often permeated with a deep sense of unity, emotional warmth, and mutual respect. Necking and petting, provided the couple are honest and sufficiently mature, can be invaluable opportunities for learning the elementary arts of love-making. The boy can reassure himself of his masculine capacity to arouse a girl; she can confirm her ability to attract and respond to the other sex. People who want to "keep sex for marriage" may be very wise and admirable if by sex they mean intercourse. But if a teenage boy or girl is fearful of *all* physical expressions of affection, the reason may be that he or she is emotionally immature and has not come to terms with the fact of sexuality. The teenager who has been impressed with strong moral ideals by his parents or church, without ever making these truly his own, may attempt to deny the existence of sexual desires, because he fears their strength and cannot integrate them with his whole personality. Difficulties in sexual adjustment in marriage may result, for a negative repudiation of the goodness of sex cannot be magically reversed on the wedding night.

However, you can easily reduce sex to a purely animal level by giving free rein to your physical desires and little thought to human sensibility. Instead of enriching relationships through necking and petting, you can isolate sex from the whole person and satisfy only your bodily needs at the expense of your partner and your self-respect. You can deny the inner conscience that tells you it is unworthy of your humanity to treat people as mere things, as instruments for your convenience. Instead of bringing two individuals closer together, petting can drive them apart, because it is used to effect a conquest of power. Instead of being a mutual discovery of the other sex, it can become a one-sided exploitation. Most frequently it is the boy who is the aggressor, trying to reassure himself of his masculinity by possessing the girl. But girls too can use their sexuality as a mere means to an end. Petting can serve as a selfish power play to get invited to a party or to gain status by dating an athlete or some other school celebrity. In such cases, instead of communicating love, petting becomes the vehicle of selfish greed.

Three things must be said about sexual behavior of this kind. In the first place, very few boys will actually force a girl into intimacy for which she is not ready. "Soft rape" or "civilized rape" *can* be resisted, though it puts a terrible burden on the girl. A girl who firmly sets a limit to petting activity can, if she wants, hold a boy to that limit—though she must also be considerate of the difficulty a boy may have in stopping the urge to orgasm past a certain level of arousal. What a boy will do, however, is to use all his persuasive powers to encourage the girl to overcome her hesitations and go along with his desires. He may try to convince her that she is lacking in femininity or sexuality, or that she is a lesbian or a freak of some kind. He may try to still her inhibitions by the use of alcohol, since (although it is more likely to reduce his sexual potency) it may offer the girl an excuse for behavior she does not really approve. But more likely the boy will affirm his undying love and devotion and plead for privileges as a proof of her affection. And this particular ploy may be very effective, for boys can be very persuasive in sensing a girl's needs and in appearing to embody just the type of masculine quality she is looking for.

Second, boys believe that girls are as easily aroused sexually as they are. They assume that because they have reached a high pitch of sexual excitement and want to proceed to orgasm, the girl must be just as fired up inside. They therefore persuade themselves that the girl who expresses hesitation about petting is only going through the motions of offering lip service to a past tradition. A boy will often tell his friends, "She asked me to stop, but I knew she didn't mean it." Few really want to pressure the girl into acting contrary to her conscience, they think it is only a matter of helping her get over the inhibitions once thought proper to women. And the boy's belief that the girl is merely acting a part has been given some support by public discussions of feminine sexuality in recent years. Reliable studies have made it clear that women are as capable of physical sexual pleasure as men, and the impression has been given (though not by the authors of the serious reports) that they want the same experience as men *at the same stage in a relationship.* In fact this is far from being the case. Advanced petting is almost always desired by a boy even if he has no real affection for the girl as a person. For her it may be repugnant if she does not sense any romantic attachment. Even if she is deeply in love with a boy, a teenage girl may not want to go that far before marriage.

Finally, most boys will respect a girl who, without being prissy and condescending, makes it clear when she has had enough or, better still, lets it be known in advance where she stands. She may not be as popular a subject for conversation in a crowd, and her name won't be passed around the school as a "good lay"; but boys may be much more interested in her as a person, and as a long-term partner. It is notable that the girls whom boys are most proud to have with them at a dance or a party are *not* the girls who have achieved a superficial popularity by giving themselves freely to all comers. Every girl has to make some decision as to which category she wants to belong to, and it's not easy.

The tragedy is that boys all too often go further than they really want to. Even the most sensitive and thoughtful boy has to deal not only with his own desires but also with the pressures of the peer group which as an impersonal mass so easily reduces sex to mere aggression. We only have to think of the terms that boys use to describe intercourse to see what the popular idea is. To think of sexual intercourse as "screwing," "laying," or "making" a girl is to reveal a sadly distorted emphasis in which the girl is not a partner in self-discovery but an object of self-assertion.

If a boy does give in to these forces which separate sex from personal values, he may become less and less capable of love or affection and eventually find it difficult to achieve any deep sexual relationship, even in marriage. Alternatively, he may find that he is less free of social or religious prohibitions than he thought, and the result may be a sense of guilt which will color his sexual attitudes and make it more difficult to enjoy open, healthy, positive sexual experiences.

The Girl's Sexual Needs

The difference between the girl's approach and that of the boy has been well stated by a British sociologist: "The boy seeks adventure while the girl looks for security." The young girl thinks of her date as a friend and companion rather than as a potential source of sexual satisfaction, and she tends to assume that he has the same attitude to her. In a study of the responses of several thousand boys and girls to various pictures of a couple sitting, standing, or running together, a significantly larger proportion of boys in the early teens assumed that the couple were emotionally and sexually involved, whereas the girls tended to see nothing more than social companionship in the relation. Only in the sixteen/seventeen age group did the two sexes come close to agreement, though even then more girls tended to think in terms of friendship than of sexual interest.

One consequence of ignorance about the difference between male and female sexuality is that the girl is often entirely unaware of the way she arouses a boy by flirting, and she may be astonished when she realizes that he is sexually excited. She may refuse him further dates because she's only interested in having a good time in a group and he wants to get her away alone in the dark. The fact that she doesn't respond is not necessarily due to the fact that she doesn't like him: she may just not be sexually aroused by a goodnight kiss or holding hands in the movies. Girls are affected by a boy's appearance, but it is his likeness to some romantic figure such as a movie star more than specific physical things like the size of his muscles or the shape of his legs that they notice. His character is likely to be just as important, and whether he is considerate and courteous on a date counts as much as his physique.

This is not to suggest at all that girls are uninterested in physical contact, such as kissing, as an expression of affection. But for many girls, petting under clothing represents the beginning of a different type of sexual intimacy. When the relationship has reached a sufficient degree of seriousness, necking or petting may be not only acceptable but very much desired. When the circumstances are right, girls are ready and able to respond to a boy's caress without embarrassment or inhibitions. A girl who has learned to respond sexually in necking and petting with her self-esteem undimmed and her trust in men confirmed is far better prepared for the physical experiences of marriage. But the context is of vital significance. Only if she believes that the boy is honestly concerned for her and if she feels some attraction to him as a whole person can most girls engage happily in sexual discovery. Only if the couple have established some communication and commitment together may she find physical intimacy meaningful. But when this stage is reached her sexual instincts may be as intense as his. Indeed it is because she seems instinctively to know that once heavy petting begins it will be difficult for her to stop that the girl hesitates to get deeply involved before she is sure of the boy's love.

It would be wrong to suggest that girls are nicely in control of every situation, any more than boys are. The pressure of the peer group is not so strongly felt, and it does not usually encourage aggressive behavior, but girls are naturally anxious to demonstrate to themselves and to their friends that they do not lack femininity. The need to feel desirable and sought after is strong. The result is that the girl may initially use her sexual charms for what is, for her, a nonsexual purpose. She may flirt with a boy or take his hand in order to start a conversation without realizing that he will assume that she has something else in mind. She wants the boy to respond to her but she expects him to be able to draw the line when she says so. As one girl put it, "You're annoyed if a boy tries to make you on the first date because it shows he thinks you're easy, and you're annoyed if he *doesn't* try to make you because it shows he doesn't fancy you."

Adjusting to Each Other's Needs

The results of the girl's ignorance about male sexuality may be as unfortunate as those of the boy's ignorance of the girl's development. A few girls quite intentionally lead boys on in order to arouse them and then frustrate their desires, but in many cases the process is unintended. However, it can be just as upsetting for the boy. He may be stimulated to the point of erection and ready for ejaculation while she is blissfully unaware of any problem. If a boy comes near to orgasm and is then expected to sip a milkshake at the drugstore counter, the effects will be nervously frustrating, and sometimes physically painful. He may conclude that the girl just doesn't like him because she won't give him what he wants—whereas she may not even know what it is that is on his mind. In some cases the experience may cause him to think girls find him unattractive, and as a result it may be difficult for him to date a girl for some time. It is important for a girl to make it clear that her lack of interest in heavy petting may not mean that she is disinterested in the boy himself.

On the other hand, if the girl goes beyond the point she feels to be appropriate, she may suffer emotionally. She may think that if a boy wants to engage in heavy petting he must mean it when he says he loves her—because she knows *she* wouldn't want it if she didn't love him. And if she finds out later that he was interested only in physical satisfaction, she may be badly hurt. She may be afraid that if she leaves him unsatisfied she will lose his affection, and she may then engage in acts that don't really have any meaning to her. The result may be that she will feel guilty or unworthy and find difficulty in future sexual encounters. I have argued that petting is in fact a healthy and helpful activity, but it can lead to profound regrets and self-condemnation if a girl discovers that she has been giving herself under false pretenses. Not a few girls acquire a deep suspicion of men and a distrust of sex because of early petting misunderstandings.

If you are to enjoy the full pleasures of sexual relationships *as a person* you have to get away from the habit of thinking about dating and petting as warfare, conquest, self-assertion, capitulation, and submission. Discovering the other sex should be a mutual activity in which each can be open, sensitive, tender, and secure. All too often the boy thinks of it as a carefully planned and cunningly executed assault on feminine virginity. All too often girls think of their bodies as citadels under attack, though they may have enticed the enemy to the very walls. Whether the boy is successful or the girl preserves herself inviolate, the operation is so centered on physical achievement that the wider range of relationships is minimized. If you are to become a mature sexual person in adulthood, you must learn that dating and petting are opportunities for sharing intimacies, mutual enrichment, developing personhood, and responsible discovery of the other sex.

5 · Who Are Gay?

There is so much publicity and discussion today about the life-styles and rights of "gays" that many teenagers have serious anxieties about their sexual orientation. It is impossible in a single chapter to deal with the issue of homosexuality in adulthood, but it is important to correct some common misunderstandings.

Homosexual means "loving one's own sex," not "loving men," and there are female homosexuals or "lesbians" as well as male. It is best to use the term for people who *in adulthood exclusively prefer to have sex with members of their own sex,* not for those who sometimes engage in homosexual acts. How many true homosexuals there are it is extremely difficult to tell—perhaps five out of a hundred among the male population and two out of a hundred among females. When homosexuals make love together, they use the same types of sexual arousal as heterosexuals do—except, of course, intercourse with the penis in the vagina. Although they cannot legally be married, many homosexuals (particularly women) live together for many years very much as a husband and wife do.

The most important thing to get straight is that there is a great difference between being a homosexual in adulthood and having homosexual desires or homosexual experiences in adolescence. Out of every hundred boys, for example, as many as fifty may have some homosexual experience during adolescence, but no more than five will probably grow up to be exclusively homosexual. The percentage for girls is much smaller. Virtually all of us are capable of experiencing sexual pleasure and even orgasm in adolescence with our own sex, but few of us are gay.

Mistaken Notions About Homosexuality

The idea that because someone engages in homosexual activity in the teens shows that person to be a homosexual is false and can be the cause of great pain. It may even lead to homosexual patterns of behavior if the individual is typed as "queer," excluded from normal social opportunities and forced into friendships only with others who are thought, or think themselves to be homosexual.

Oversimplified ideas about what is "appropriate" behavior for a boy or girl may also lead to the mistaken assumption that someone is permanently homosexual. The girl who is always being called a "tomboy" because she likes climbing trees or playing football, or the boy who is called "sissy" because he enjoys painting or wants to be a ballet dancer may begin to wonder about their sexual identities. They may hesitate to date members of the other sex, or feel inadequate about their sexual roles. In fact their preferences for play or their plans for a profession have nothing whatever to do with their being homosexual.

It is vital to know that during adolescence a homosexual phase is quite normal (though not universal) and the fact that a boy enjoys physical intimacy with another boy, or a girl with a girl, is insignificant unless it becomes the cause of unnecessary guilt or anxiety. We have seen that masturbation is, particularly for boys, a normal part of the process of self-discovery—an exploration and affirmation of one's sexual powers. We have also seen how important it is for the teenager to move out of the childhood role as a member of the family toward self-identity. And we have noted the importance of the peer group as a support for the individual as he or she breaks away from parental dependence to become a person with a distinct identity and integral values. But at first the peer group is almost always a homosexual group. A boy's pals with whom he first identifies himself over against the family unit are boys, and a girl's friends are at first other girls. Inevitably, therefore, the business of discovering genital sexuality during puberty and early adolescence often includes mutual handling and exploration of the sex organs. Inevitably also, because puberty brings with it the initial urge toward love for people outside the family circle, relationships with one's close friends of the same sex often have something of the intensity of later love for a member of the other sex. It is consistent with the difference between boys and girls that we noted in the previous chapter that male homosexual associations tend to be more genital and less emotional, while adolescent girls develop absorbing "crushes" on other girls or female teachers. But these passionate feminine relationships are just as sexual (and usually just as temporary). While adolescent girls are less likely to engage in any genital contact, the physical element in their love is expressed more publicly in kissing and hugging, which our society happens to find acceptable between women and not between men.

Two Results of Ignorance

Out of sheer ignorance, however, many boys and some girls who experience homosexual contacts leading to orgasm, or even merely homosexual desires, suspect that they are finally and permanently homosexual in orientation. Because our society has for so long condemned homosexuals, the boy or girl who finds adolescent homosexual experience pleasurable inevitably feels a sense of guilt. Religious teaching, which has interpreted the story of God's destruction of the city of Sodom in the book of Genesis (chapter 19) as a condemnation of homosexuality, encourages the fear that this is an especially horrible perversion. Boys often begin to harbor profound fears about their own masculinity. Instead of recognizing this as a normal stage of sexual self-discovery, they fear that they are less than fully male. If their first attempts at dating girls prove unsatisfactory, they are likely to assume (quite wrongly) that it is because they lack the necessary manly qualities. As a result, instead of moving easily from the homosexual phase to the heterosexual stage of discovering the other sex, they may be hesitant and lacking in self-confidence. Girls need to be aware of this, and sensitive to the possible need of their dates for encouragement and reassurance about their masculinity.

Another equally unfortunate fallacy is that there exists a particular homosexual type of physique. Thus, boys of slight build and girls who are more muscular are popularly suspected of being homosexual. A boy whose penis is smaller than others, or who is late in developing body hair, often fears quite unnecessarily that he is abnormal. Boys who show signs of breast enlargement can be terribly worried because they do not know that this is a common and usually temporary side-effect of puberty. Girls may be concerned because their figures are too boyish, because they are as tall as their male classmates, or because they don't find the physical aspects of dating very pleasant in the early teens. But all these are false alarms. Many of them are due to the irregularity of each individual's growth at puberty. There is no sound evidence that homosexuals are distinguishable by particular physical characteristics.

Encounters With Adult Homosexuals

Some teenagers are approached or "propositioned" by adult homosexuals. Nobody is likely to be permanently affected by an isolated experience, and there is no evidence that homosexuals are more likely to accost young children than heterosexuals. But such individuals should be reported because the law quite rightly protects the young from molestation, and a deviant sexual encounter is often frightening and can be harmful. On the other hand, there is no cause for panic. The idea that homosexuals "know their own" and that because you have been solicited you have some external or internal mark of homosexual leanings is nonsense. It cannot be sufficiently emphasized that even if you find the experience physically enjoyable this is no indication of permanent homosexuality.

Of course, the possibility that an individual will grow up as a homosexual remains. As we have seen, perhaps one in ten of those boys who have homosexual experience in the teens turns out to be an adult homosexual. In some cases there are probably biological and physical factors that make this unavoidable—though it's not the end of the world if it happens. Some homosexual adults believe that they knew from an early age where their sexual interests lay. But it is probably the fact that some homosexuals could have developed differently if they had received proper advice and treatment during adolescence. Many experts think that early childhood experiences make heterosexual development difficult, and that these can be identified and treated with professional help. Any boy or girl who finds that by the late teens homosexual interests and activities are increasing and heterosexual desires are absent should certainly talk to a doctor or psychiatrist. In the modern world they are likely to be sympathetic and helpful rather than condemnatory or rejecting.

Why Not Be A Homosexual?

But the questions may well be asked, "Why bother to change if you find homosexual behavior satisfying and preferable to contacts with the other sex?" "Isn't it out of date to regard homosexuality as a disease to be cured, and aren't many homosexuals entirely happy with their way of life?" To discuss these issues would require a book of its own, and I can only say here that there is a great difference between the advice experts would give to an adult and to a teenager. It is probably true that an attempt to alter radically the sexual orientation of many older homosexuals would be pointless. The individual's habits and patterns of response have probably become too fixed to respond to treatment. And because in our society homosexuals are forced to organize their lives around their sexual contacts, a "change" might threaten a person's whole social role and relationships. But this does not mean that it will make little difference whether you grow up a heterosexual or a homosexual.

In the first place, while it is generally agreed that homosexuality is not a sickness or a personality disorder, it does reflect an inability to develop part of one's sexual potential. It is quite true that many homosexuals have played, and are playing constructive roles in society. Many live stable, integrated, and happy lives. Some perhaps develop creative gifts and loving human relationships that might have been denied to them (and to the rest of the world) had they not been homosexual. But it is still true that they are unable to enjoy the self-enlargement that is open to us through sexual relations with those whose sexual makeup is complementary to

ours. And they are denied the privilege (and the pain) of
parenthood.

Second, on the quite practical level, our society still im-
poses legal and social penalties on homosexuals and three
out of every four Americans disapprove of homosexual
relations. Homosexuals are unhappily liable to blackmail
and to discrimination in jobs and housing. They are
sometimes the object of bitterness and violence—probably
from men who have hidden doubts about their own sexuality. I think all of this totally wrong, and I support those
groups working for full gay rights. But there's no point in
choosing to be the object of social rejection. When many
homosexuals were asked, "If you had a son, would you
want him to be a homosexual?" only two out of every
hundred said, "Yes."

In short, don't assume you are gay because you have
sexual experience with a member of your own sex. If you
fail, during your teens, to develop an interest in the other
sex do talk to some competent professional about it. If
you eventually grow up homosexual, don't be ashamed of
what you are but make your sexual relationships as rich
and mature as you can.

CAMROSE LUTHERAN COLLEGE
LIBRARY

6 · Sex and Society

(Our society's traditional view of sex is quite simple: intercourse should be engaged in only by people who are married to each other. Many teenagers think the idea quite unrealistic even if they approve of it in principle. Others would argue that to refrain from sexual intercourse until marriage is actually harmful or stupid. We shall discuss these objections in later chapters. For the present, however, let's look at the public sexual code, and see what can be said in its favor.)

Official Attitudes Toward Premarital Sex

We should start by distinguishing the official ideal from actual practice. Sexual intercourse outside of marriage is illegal in more than two-thirds of the states of the Union. But this legal prohibition on premarital intercourse does not reflect actual practice. A majority of the population engages, at some time, in this behavior, even though it is strictly criminal. More than half of the population, according to a 1978 study, think that sex before marriage is not always wrong. Nor is this discrepancy between official ideals and actual practice anything new. There has never been a time when anything like 100 percent of the population has conformed to the letter of the law in sexual conduct.

On the other hand, it is absurd to assume that because a lot of people act contrary to the standards upheld publicly by our society, these standards are necessarily out of date or misguided. A great many people tell lies, steal things from stores, cheat the income-tax authorities, and have automobile wrecks; but most of them would not want the principles of truthfulness, honesty, and respect for human life to be abandoned wholesale. They may complain when they get caught, but they realize that if our society gave up expecting people to act responsibly, and failed to punish the more obvious offenders, life would become chaotic. As one famous philosopher put it, we have to judge our own individual acts by considering what would happen if everybody else did the same. If you do this you may not always act consistently, but you will think twice before throwing overboard all the sexual standards upheld in our society.

You may find it hard to think in terms of the long-term future, but you have to face the likelihood that you will grow up to live as an adult in a society more or less continuous with the present. And whatever changes may be desirable in the *form* of family life we know, there are values in it that most people would not want to lose. One is the right of women to love and be loved as equals. Another is the security and affection a child gets from its parents. Something like our pattern of monogamy and family identity seems to be essential to the preservation of these elements. And undoubtedly one of the major factors tending to sustain marriage in our culture has been the tradition that a husband and wife share the special intimacy of sexual union with each other alone. It is still true, despite greater freedom in sexual behavior, that *the majority of people who have intercourse before they are married do so only with the person they eventually marry.* Thus premarital intercourse is more often an anticipation of marriage than a repudiation of it. The view that intercourse should be a special bond between a man and a woman is still accepted by the majority, even if the union is often established before the formal ceremony of marriage.

The Effects of Sexual Freedom on Our Society

But what will be the effect if all restrictions on sexual freedom are removed? If people become accustomed to intercourse quite apart from any formal marriage bond, will it continue to hold them together after marriage? Why should the habits of adolescence be suddenly set aside and those who have enjoyed sex with several partners become faithful husbands and wives? Will not the result be an increasing number of broken homes and a multiplication of personal and sexual problems in the succeeding generation? These are questions to which no decisive answer can be given in advance. But there is obviously some justification for the anxiety expressed in them. And only a very self-centered or short-sighted person will ignore the good of society as a whole in working out his or her own standards of sexual behavior.

Can A Religious View of Sex Be Healthy?

It is, of course, religious tradition that most firmly holds that sexual intercourse should be reserved for marriage. And religious overtones are almost always present in any discussion of sex. When I once asked a group of teenagers what they would like to discuss on an educational program, one of the first questions was, "Is sex always sinful?" Even those who have little religious conviction of their own are still often deeply influenced by the persistence in our culture of moral ideals based on the Bible. Basic to this is the commandment, "Thou shalt not commit adultery," and the strong condemnation in the New Testament of "fornication." As a matter of fact the commandment does not mention sexual intercourse between *unmarried* persons. And "fornication" originally referred to sexual activity in a context very different than that which prevails today. The personal love and friendship we often take for granted outside marriage was quite unknown in biblical times. Any sexual intimacy before marriage would almost certainly have been of the purely impersonal kind that exists between a prostitute and the customer to whom she sells her body. Whether Saint Paul, for example, would have regarded all premarital intercourse as *equally* sinful if he had lived today is open to question. But in any case, official Jewish and Christian teaching still firmly holds that intercourse outside marriage is wrong.

The basis of this position is the belief that the physical union of intercourse brings two people together in a special way as "one flesh." Whether we recognize it or not, what we do with our body involves our whole personality. For those united in marriage with God's blessing and help, according to religious teaching, sex can contribute to their mutual good. But if the physical act is isolated from the obligations of lifelong commitment, it becomes a kind of lie, a pretense, a false giving of the body because the whole self is not shared. If we engage in intercourse apart from love and the intention to live together in marriage, we deny or destroy something of our humanity, according to the teaching of most religious bodies.

Unfortunately, this recognition of the value of sex as an expression of love was soon lost in Christianity, and the Church tended to be suspicious of or hostile to the sexual side of man's nature. Celibacy was exalted as a superior form of Christian service (an idea now widely questioned even in Catholic circles) and medieval theologians taught that even married couples were better

Christians if they avoided intercourse except strictly for reproduction. Luther and Calvin had a more positive appreciation of sex, but they too believed that married couples should avoid sexual pleasure as far as they could. It wasn't until the Second Vatican Council (1965) that the Catholic Church declared that the sexual expression of love in marriage is "decent and worthy" and signifies a mutual giving by which a married couple "with joyful and grateful spirit reciprocally enrich each other."

The deeply rooted religious anxiety about sex is still with us, however. If we say of someone that he's "living in sin," we know quite well what is meant. It never occurs to us that the sin referred to might be extortion, pride, or racial prejudice. When someone is described as "immoral," we immediately suspect her of sexual weakness, never of greed, jealousy, brutality or arrogance. Christian teaching has implanted in our cultural conscience not only a positive appreciation of marriage but also a negative distaste for sex. Many Catholic authorities still teach children that any sexual pleasure outside of marriage is sinful. A Protestant theologian states dogmatically: "Before marriage it is best to keep every sort of sexual excitement toward your fiancée under complete control, since it is not good for her." Judaism has maintained a more positive attitude to sex, regarding intercourse as a religious duty within marriage, but an official publication of the Union of Orthodox Jewish Congregations of America tells young readers that all physical contact, *including holding hands,* should be avoided before marriage, because it brings into play forces the average person cannot cope with.

This negative attitude had a great deal of influence until recently because it was supported by the threats and fears of pregnancy and disease. We know now that there is no divinely ordained connection between premarital intercourse and pregnancy or venereal disease. These are still real risks (see chapter 8), but religious authorities who have relied on fear to support their teaching are widely discredited among teenagers.

A boy or girl who remains virginal simply because of fear of hell-fire is not doing anything particularly admirable. To follow any moral teaching simply because you are frightened of the consequences of ignoring it is never a mature thing to do, either as an adult or as an adolescent. But the fact that certain ideas have been supported by bad arguments, or enforced by false threats, does not show that they are wrong in themselves. In adolescence one has to move from the childhood acceptance of values merely on authority to the acceptance of them because they are seen to be true or good in themselves. You have to decide which, if any, of society's ideas of sex make sense to you. And it would be as childish to reject all these ideas simply because they have been taught you as religious dogma as it would be to continue holding them simply because you first learnt them from your parents or church. And this may mean that the Christian or Jewish idea of marriage does become an integral part of your own values. There is nothing immature or childish in choosing premarital chastity because of a deeply held religious conviction about the nature of sexual union and its relation to marriage, provided it's your own conviction.

Studies of contemporary sexual behavior show quite consistently that those with strong religious faith much more frequently avoid premarital intercourse than those without. Those whose sexual restraint is based on a realistic and conscious decision to preserve the intimacy of intercourse for the one person with whom they share married life cannot be dismissed as mere conformists. Religious faith is often the source and center of great personal integrity and healthy relationships. When someone exercises sexual restraint out of love rather than law, and preserves his or her chastity for positive reasons rather than out of fear, there is no basis for questioning the maturity of the person's sexual development.

Social Contradictions

The distorted denial of the goodness of sex is being gradually corrected in religious circles. But its effects are still present in the public attitudes of our society. There are laws in several states forbidding many petting practices if the girl is under twenty-one, *even if she consents.* Touching the genitals of the other sex can bring a person a sentence of ten years in Indiana or Wyoming. Teenagers in some states can find themselves in court as "juvenile delinquents" for petting in a movie theater or a car. Whatever we may think of these laws, and however little they may be enforced, it is only sensible to recognize that they exist, and that they reflect the continued unrealistic suspicion of sex in America.

An exaggerated fear of sexuality touches all our lives in the censorship—both legal and informal—imposed by our society on literature, movies, and television. And the effect of long-standing taboos about sex is all too often that young people are given little or no help in establishing responsible, honest, and meaningful sexual standards for themselves.

For example, children are very much aware that adults regard certain "four-letter words" as "dirty." But it is mere chance that several of the common words connected with sex in our language happen to have four letters. *Love* and *work* are in the same category. There is nothing about certain combinations of consonants and vowels that makes them "dirty" in themselves: it is purely the usage to which they are put and the associations they carry that make them publicly unacceptable. The words *bloody* and *bugger,* for example, were until very recently taboo in Britain, but they have never been regarded as objectionable in polite speech in America. The word *cunt* was used in the seventeenth century as a technical term for the vagina without any suggestions of vulgarity. What is important is the cumulative effect of such language on the sexual atmosphere of our society. Most of the four-letter words have associations of violence which can subtly color our whole sexual outlook. The way sexual terms are used for *nonsexual* acts of cruelty or exploitation makes this very clear. "Fuck you" is a verbal assault with overtones of aggression which tells us a good deal about the user's view of intercourse. "I got screwed" means "I was swindled or exploited"—and that's just how some men view woman's sexual role.

The sooner we get away from avoiding or using particular terms simply because they happen to be slang words for sexual acts or sexual organs, the better. What we need to examine is the emotional context and the psychological attitude expressed or encouraged by four-letter words. If we habitually speak and think of sex aggressively and impersonally, it may be much more difficult to develop truly personal loving sexual relationships.

Pornography

Our laws and conventions about "dirty" pictures and books are equally confused and confusing. By concentrating attention on the question of nudity, our society has distorted the whole issue. There was recently a newspaper headline, "Police Chase 'Nudes' on Quayside"; but it appeared on reading the report that the fuss was not about the overexposure of human bodies, only about pictures. Some waste paper being imported into Britain from Sweden for pulp had been scattered by the wind and out-of-date pinups had been strewn all over the place. Police, customs officials, and security men had arrived in force to put an end to the excitement. That the nude female body should be on view, even on paper, was horrifying to officialdom in Britain, as it would be in America. But the idea that the human body is in itself disgusting is a by-product of the negative antisexualism which has so affected our culture. We tend to blame the Puritans or the Victorians for this, but while they certainly contributed to it, it is worth remembering that it was a medieval pope who put panties on the nudes in Michelangelo's painting of the Last Judgment. At other times, both before and since, great artists and sculptors have freely portrayed the human body (pubic hair and genitals included) without any sense of indecency. A Greek statue of a perfect male or female form does not arouse sexual lust but only honest delight and admiration. It is largely because society has labeled the naked body indecent that sexual arousal is derived from photographs or peeping in windows. Most boys soon get over this fascination (girls seldom feel any need to look for naked men), and I suspect that displays of pinups are often nothing more than an affirmation of the goodness of sex in contrast to adult suspicion and prudery.

The question of books or photographs describing sexual acts or deviations is more complex and controversial. It is still widely held that such literature triggers violent behavior. But many authorities have become convinced that people with the tendency to commit rape or other crimes are likel / to find substitute satisfaction in reading pornographic materials; thus their aggressive tendencies may be defused by sexual fantasies. Probably there is some truth in both arguments. In some cases a person with a disposition toward sexual perversion may be stimulated to antisocial acts by reading a book or magazine. But censorship gives an additional aura of excitement to illicit trash, doesn't seem to reduce the flow of obscene books, and always threatens the work of serious and respected authors. If our culture had a more healthy attitude to sexuality, provided its young with better education about sex, and removed the attraction of "forbidden fruit," it is likely (to judge from the experience of the Scandinavian countries) that much of the problem would solve itself.

On the other hand, many psychiatrists recognize that damage can be done to the sexual development of some children if they are subjected to obscene material before they have the emotional capacity to recognize its inadequacies and distortions. This is particularly true if sex is associated with violence, aggression, and sadistic pleasure. What is wanted, I believe, is a law which will make it difficult for children to buy sexually distorted material. This will not prevent their reading it, but will make clear that responsible adults reject the exaggerated, impersonal, and purely physical use of sex. If young people are protected from public displays or pandering of obscenity and encounter it only when they have acquired some standards of judgment and maturity, it is unlikely that it will do much harm. By the late teens most are capable of evaluating pornography for what it is.

The Influence of Movies and TV

Finally, we must briefly consider the way in which movies and television affect sexual attitudes. Here again there seems to be a confusion between sexuality, which is a good and healthy element in human life, and sexual behavior, which may be mature and loving or may be merely aggressive and selfish. On the whole our society has been at pains to deny adolescents any opportunity to see the human body naked and to censor scenes of lovemaking beyond the first stage of kissing or embracing. The clear impression left by this policy is that somehow these things are objectionable or degrading *in them-*

selves—a perpetuation of the negative attitude to sex we have already noted. On the other hand, you grow up with the apparently acceptable idea that any manly figure like Agent 007 can freely enjoy a roll in the hay with any women he wants. It is clear that James Bond and his type epitomize an ideal which allows men to achieve sexual satisfaction with every attractive woman they meet on the basis of purely physical response. It is equally clearly implied that any girl worth her femininity is ready to be turned on like a television set (and is equally untroubled when she is abruptly turned off!). The girl at first resists, but when the hero overpowers her, her inhibitions drop away as easily as her clothing. The code does not allow you to see her naked body, but it does allow you to absorb (with adult approval and sponsorship!) a view of sexual relationships which is purely physical and impersonal and an image of feminine sexuality which is distorted and impoverished.

Once again, the value of censorship is doubtful. Efforts to prevent impressionable young children from thinking that violence can solve every problem, including sexual needs, are certainly desirable. But to restrict movies on the basis that they portray nudity while allowing them to depict violence is to leave the important questions unanswered or even unasked. What happens when certain movies are restricted to "adult audiences" is that some teenagers go to them looking for mere titillation—and that is what they tend to find. Because they approach the movie with distorted expectations, the real depth and significance of the story may be missed. What we need is an honest public acceptance of sexuality which makes no secret of its importance and pleasure, but challenges us to recognize its complexity.

7 · Does Love Make It Right?

A few years ago a Canadian sociologist predicted in a public lecture that romantic love had reached the end of its evolution and would soon be obsolete. On the other hand, an English TV interviewer who talked to many adults and teenagers came to the conclusion that while the forms of romance change, its basic quality remains. She found that despite the widespread rejection by today's teenagers of the dreams of romance that inspired their parents, adolescents are just as likely to fall in love as they ever were. Many teenagers ridicule the idea that they are destined for one particular member of the other sex forever. The "knight in shining armor" image or the picture of the girl in virginal white being showered with rose petals seems pretty corny to most teens. If romance means finding "Miss Right" with whom you can live happily ever after in a country cottage (or a split-level suburban home), few boys are interested. If falling in love means being swept off your feet by a movie idol like Rudolph Valentino with shiny slicked hair who desires you passionately but treats you like fragile porcelain, today's girls are too sophisticated to be candidates. But if it's a matter of deep, all-consuming devotion to one particular boy or girl, this generation is as much involved emotionally as any earlier one. One teenager speaks of love as "a magnetism between us" and says "If I lost her I'd sort of die, I'd go mad. . . . If I search for years, a million years, I'd never find anyone like her. She's all I live for, all I work for." A sampling of the current pop tunes will show that most of the lyrics are about love. It's no longer assumed that you fall in love only once and then forever. Fewer and fewer teenagers think that all sexual intimacy should be preserved (even in theory) for the wedding night and the honeymoon. But most of them expect and hope that they will sooner or later meet someone they will want to share their whole lives and bodies with, someone who will satisfy their ideal of companionship and inspire their unqualified devotion, someone they can trust and be trusted by without fear or reservation. We know instinctively that there's a different quality to this relationship—like the eighth-grader who was asked on a TV show if she'd ever been in love and replied, "No—and I haven't even been in like."

On the other hand, it's not always easy to distinguish between being in love and infatuation—literally, "infoolishness." One of Shakespeare's characters says cynically, "Love is merely a madness." The very term *"falling in love"* suggests an experience over which we have no control, and the boy or girl in love is often beyond any rational discussion of the imperfections of the beloved. A sociologist has affirmed that the conception of love held by high school students is "almost completely sentimental . . . protective and yummy." Certainly romantic love alone is an inadequate basis for marriage, as we shall see in the next chapter.

Falling in Love

But at the same time falling in love or being in love is an experience which enriches your life, quickens your heart, arouses your deepest instincts, and at least to some extent lifts you out of your self-centeredness and isolation. As one psychiatrist has pointed out, the capacity of lovers to see more in each other than other people can be a distortion which is dangerous if it is not checked and balanced by some recognition of actual weaknesses; but at the same time it may reflect a more acute and penetrating perception of the unrealized potentialities and strengths of the partner. While it is important to recognize the limitations of romantic love, then, it should also be welcomed as the starting point of the deepest human relationship—the union of two persons in mutual self-giving commitment. At first in love you are most aware of what the other person has to give. As love grows you become more and more concerned about what you have to give to and share with him or her. Mature love, as Erich Fromm put it in his famous book *The Art of Loving,* is "essentially an act of will, of decision to commit my life completely to that of one other person." When you love deeply, you no longer desire to control or possess another human being; you are concerned, in Fromm's words, with care, responsibility, respect, and union. You do not need to weave make-believe dreams about the one you love; you can face the facts and still want to share your lives together.

There is, of course, no necessary connection between sex and love in this deep sense. It is quite possible to engage in sexual intimacy with someone you hardly know, about whom you care nothing, or even whom you dislike as a person. Lust, rather than love, may motivate your sexual behavior. You may be interested only in satisfying your own physical needs without any thought for the integrity or good of the other individual involved.

But despite the fears of some adults it appears that few adolescents find the divorce of sex from love satisfying or acceptable. Although many teenagers reject the traditional standard of premarital chastity as a rigid rule, and are quite happy to enjoy sex up to and including inter-course outside of the marriage bond, the number who are promiscuous is small. Promiscuity is the engagement in sexual activity on a purely transient basis and without any affection for or interest in the partner, and while un-doubtedly some adolescent sex is of this quality, few are satisfied with it or happy with themselves when they act that way. Some men and women (the Don Juans and the nymphomaniacs) develop patterns of sexual behavior of this impersonal, irresponsible type, but psychiatrists regard them as emotionally sick in adulthood. "Men and women," wrote Erich Fromm, "who devote their lives to unrestricted sexual satisfaction do not attain happiness, and very often suffer from neurotic conflicts or symp-toms. The complete satisfaction of all instinctual needs is not only not a basis for happiness, it does not even guar-antee sanity."

Fortunately such unhappy people are uncommon, and they need our compassion and sympathy rather than re-jection. Anyone in late adolescence who fears that he or she is incapable of deep and satisfying sexual relation-ships should seek professional help. The great major-ity feel that the more intimate sexual acts, particularly intercourse, are really meaningful and enjoyable only within the context of love. "Love makes it right, so long as nobody gets hurt" is a frequent defense. "As a casual thing sex is wrong," wrote a girl of seventeen in reply to a questionnaire. "Kids who regard it as a fun-filled evening disgust me."

Does Love Make it Right?

The difficulties arise, however, when you try to apply the high moral principle that love makes it right to specific situations. Sex may not necessarily involve love, but ro-mantic love inevitably involves sex in some shape or form.

I don't mean intercourse: as we've seen, it is a fundamental mistake to suppose that sex occurs only when a couple go to bed together. When a boy and girl find themselves in love, the formal exchanges of earlier dating practices—kissing and necking—take on a new dimension and a new urgency. The powerful sexual urge, particularly of the boy whose sexual drive reaches its highest point in the late teens, tends to impel a couple into ever more heavy petting. Sexual arousal is stimulated by talk and example among the peer group, and adults play their part in complicating the situation by the use of sex for commercial purposes in advertising and on TV and movie screens. The question "How far should you go?" becomes difficult to answer and even more difficult to observe in practice. The crucial question for many teenagers is: Does love justify intercourse?

The answer is, surely, that it does: but love is a word that covers a wide range of emotions and relationships, and the question is better expressed thus: At what point is love sufficiently strong and deep to justify intercourse? Underlying the dating pattern is the assumption that certain types of sexual intimacy are appropriate to certain situations. A girl who will go to bed with a boy on the first date is pretty universally regarded as a tramp: in fact, she is emotionally sick. However widely local patterns of dating, going steady, pinning, or whatever vary, they all imply that certain degrees of personal knowledge or affection normally precede different stages of physical contact—and various stages of more or less exclusive association with one particular boy or girl. In the early teens dating is much freer than it is later, but the extent to which a couple share physical contact in this type of casual encounter is limited. Then, as you begin to narrow the field of people with whom you feel comfortable and spend more time with one boy or girl, you share more of your body as well as more of your social, emotional, or religious interests. At the same time you tend to restrict your sexual activities more and more to one person. Eventually you find yourself really in love, and one particular boy or girl becomes "all I live for, all I work for." At this point it seems to some that intercourse is a natural and justifiable expression of love. Having found the one person whom you want to be with every day and with whom you feel you can share every problem and every joy, why not share the special sexual experience of intercourse? Since there already exists a unity of spirit and love between you, why hestitate to establish full unity of body? Finally, since intercourse is uniquely enjoyable, why deny oneself this pleasure?

I have a great deal of sympathy with teenagers who feel that their love should find expression here and now in sexual union. I do not think intercourse before marriage is degrading or terribly sinful, provided it expresses concern and respect between two people. And I do not think it necessarily harmful to the relationship of the couple concerned or to their eventual happiness. But I do believe that young people need to be aware of facts and implications about intercourse which they often learn only when it is too late to turn the clock back.

First, a couple of facts which anyone should take seriously. Nowadays it is very much out of style, quite rightly, to use the threat of venereal disease or pregnancy as a means of enforcing chastity. But it is important that teenagers in making their own decisions about sexual activity should know what the dangers are and take them into account. Certainly anyone who talks about "love making it right" should consider the possible consequences that may result from going all the way. So hear this:

1. Venereal diseases are *not* under control by modern drugs, they *are* contracted from dates and steadies (not only from pickups and prostitutes), and syphilis and

herpes *can* be transmitted by other means than intercourse. The basic facts are given in chapter 8, and all that needs to be said here is that *if you engage in sexual intercourse with anyone who has done so with a third party you run a good chance of contracting a venereal disease.* Equally, of course, if *you* have been with another person who might have VD (and may not know it, or may not have told you), you can very easily infect the person you claim to love.

2. Despite the availability of birth control methods, over a million teenagers in the United States become pregnant every year. Most of the girls who have illegitimate babies have been going steady with or been engaged to the father of the child, and most of them believed themselves to be in love when they conceived. It is usually *not* the promiscuous or irresponsible boy or girl who slips up but the couple who intend to exercise self-control, take no precautions in advance, and get carried away by the atmosphere of a romantic evening. Carelessness, ignorance, and the ineffective use of contraceptives are extremely common among teenagers. Many girls have totally inaccurate ideas about the "safe period," supposing it to be about the middle of their monthly cycle, when that is actually the most likely time to conceive. Boys tend to assume that every girl is "on the pill," and they seldom understand that to be effective this means careful and regular use for twenty-one days every month.

Many girls disastrously underestimate the consequences of pregnancy out of marriage. Some, as we have noted, think that having a baby will establish their identities as women. Some just like the idea of having a human doll to play with. Some suppose that getting pregnant will ensure that their boyfriend sticks with them. Some assume, unfairly and wrongly, that they can dump the baby on their own mother or an elder sister. But the reality is very different. Most teenagers who get pregnant drop out of school, enter into marriages that soon fail, or find themselves on welfare and without hope of finding a job. Teenage mothers attempt suicide seven times as often as other girls of their age.

One thing love certainly doesn't make right is having an unwanted child. The responsibility for avoiding that tragedy is at least as much the boy's as the girl's. Indeed, since he is going to suffer less from the results of carelessness than the girl, any boy who argues for intercourse on the basis of love has an obvious duty to read and act on the information given in the next chapter.

Can You Know It's Love?

Provided you've taken precautions, though, what is there against expressing your love in the deepest way sexually? The basic difficulty is that it is extremely hard for any teenage couple to know with any real certainty that their love is strong and real enough to justify sharing together the ultimate intimacy of intercourse. It is a sheer matter of statistical fact that the great majority of experiences of falling in love in the teens do *not* turn out to be permanent, however final and perfect the relationship may seem at the time. However hard it may be to recognize the fact, the likelihood is that the first or second or third time you fall head over heels in love in your teens will not be the last. If you engage in sexual intercourse on the basis that "love makes it right" because *this* is the love of your life, and this girl or this boy the *one* person you can share your body with, you are very likely to be wrong. For the firm evidence shows that in all probability he or she is nothing of the kind, and in this case if you do go ahead and engage in full sexual union together, there will be nothing special with which to express your unique relationship to the boy or girl you eventually do share your whole life with in marriage. If intercourse is the

most profound and wonderful experience of love between two people, it seems logical to preserve it for the
person with whom you share the unity of marriage. For
love is not complete until you actually take the step of
committing yourself for life. Love makes it right, but love
is more than feeling or talk; love sufficient to justify the
final intimacy of sexual union surely includes the readiness to share your future with a particular man or
woman. Every time you have intercourse with another
person you reduce the significance and quality of the act
as a bond linking you uniquely and exclusively with one
person. As Dr. Mary Calderone asked in an article in
Redbook magazine, "How many times, and how casually,
are you willing to invest a portion of your total self, and
to be the custodian of a like investment from the other
person without the sureness of knowing that these in-
vestments are being made for keeps?"

There are special difficulties in applying the high-
sounding principle "Love makes it right" during the
teens. We have seen in earlier chapters that the process of
sexual development, the establishment of independent
self-identity, and the discovery of the other sex are inex-
tricably intertwined during adolescence. The result is that
an adolescent finds it virtually impossible to distinguish
the need for personal growth and achievement from the
ability to love another person. We have seen that falling
in love can be the beginning of mature, self-giving love.
But the achievement of love that can survive the tests of
disappointment, sickness, or disagreement takes time and
effort.

All too few adults learn to love profoundly and unsel-
fishly. And while some teenage experiences of love develop into permanent relationships, the great majority of
early intense attachments to a member of the other sex
are motivated by unconscious needs which are basically
self-concerned. This is not to say that every boy or girl

who swears undying devotion is being insincere. Consciously he or she means every word of it, but in fact something much more complicated and misleading is going on. For example, a boy who appeals to a girl to sleep with him may think he loves her deeply, while actually he is using her to demonstrate to himself or his friends his capacity to "score." The real test of his sincerity comes when the girl replies, "If you really love me, you won't try to pressure me into something I'm not ready for." Love, if it is deep and sincere, must surely be concerned about the needs and preferences of the partner as much as about its own satisfaction. Unless the boy cares about the girl enough to forego the price of sexual conquest for her sake, the maturity of his love is in question.

The Girl's Special Problems

On the other hand, a girl who believes herself to have found the one man with whom she can share her whole life may actually be responding out of loneliness to the first male figure in her life who has ever shown her any affection and is now filling the gap left by an absent or withdrawn father in childhood. She may think she is eternally in love with him, whereas she is in reality only temporarily fascinated by having a man to care for her. One study of teenage sex behavior found that many of the girls had engaged in sexual intercourse because they were insecure and attributed this to a lack of parental love. One high school junior said, "Most girls I know who have premarital affairs get little or no affection at home, and falsely think any boy who wants a sexual relationship feels love for them."

As we have seen earlier, in chapter 4, the attitude of girls towards sexual intimacy in the teens is very different from that of boys. Even when a girl in her late teens becomes seriously attached to a boy, she may not share his enthusiasm for intercourse outside of marriage, nor does she necessarily feel the same need for sexual satisfaction in orgasm. In the teens the sexual needs of a girl are often adequately met by being together with a boy, sharing his interests and social life, and enjoying the less intimate contacts of necking and petting.

By the age of twelve, nine out of ten American girls have decided that they want to get married eventually, and the possible consequences of casual sex are never far from their minds. Intercourse, even when precautions have been taken against pregnancy (not always, as we have seen, successfully), is still for the girl the act which connotes motherhood rather than (as it is for the boy) the act which leads to sexual release in orgasm. It has been said that for the woman the sexual act is not a consummation but a beginning. She is usually concerned that any child she might bear should be provided with security and parental care. She is therefore unlikely to give herself happily and enthusiastically to a boy unless she feels that there exists some relationship between them of permanence and commitment.

Of course, it is not very difficult for a boy to persuade her that this is the case: he may well believe it himself. If her own sexual instincts are strong and she wants to sleep with him, she may persuade herself that it must be love because "nice" girls are only aroused by the real thing. If she is basically unexcited by the prospect but likes the boy and wants to enjoy his company, she may overcome her hesitations by arguing thus: "I don't particularly want this experience, but it seems to mean so much to him that I'll go along. If I wanted so desperately to go to bed with someone, I'd love him terribly—so when he says he loves me he must mean it. I like him enough, and there's no danger if we're careful, so maybe it's worth it if it pleases him and draws us closer." Unfortunately, the chances are that the actual experience won't draw them together.

The Effects of Early Intercourse

Undoubtedly there are cases in which intercourse is a profoundly meaningful experience for a teenage couple who are mature enough to give themselves to each other in love. I do not believe that premarital intercourse is necessarily selfish or exploitative. But the indications are that few couples of high school age find it either "right" or beneficial to their relationship.

A survey of psychiatrists reported in 1979 showed that very few of them thought that most teenagers *between the ages of sixteen to nineteen* were capable of making a mature decision to engage in sexual relations. The majority thought that sexual experience usually increased the confusions and conflicts of adolescence, rather than contributing to growth and self-confidence. Contrary to widespread myth *there is no scientific evidence to prove that premarital intercourse leads to successful marriage.* While couples who have abstained from intercourse may be slower to achieve mutual sexual satisfaction, they may be better able to develop full and permanent personal relationships in marriage.

While the boy is likely to enjoy orgasm in any circumstances, the physical experience is often unsatisfying for the girl. There are times when the boy is insensitive or so highly aroused that the girl's hymen is broken violently. All too often it turns out that once a boy has enjoyed his orgasm he is uninterested in the girl's needs—or mistakenly assumes that she has "come" at the same time. The conditions under which teenagers have intercourse are often cramped and secretive. A girl who is fearful or anxious and unable to relax freely is unlikely to enjoy the experience. The Kinsey report found that girls who have unsatisfying or painful experiences of intercourse premaritally often have serious difficulties in adjusting to sexual fulfillment in marriage.

It is true that the greater sexual freedom of the past few years, with its recognition of the fact that women can properly enjoy sexual pleasure as much as men, has led to a reduction of the number of girls who find their first experience of intercourse painful or embarrassing. But emotional distress and self-contempt are not uncommon. Girls are much more likely than boys to have religious or moral objections to intercourse before marriage, and if these objections are overridden by pressure from the boy or rationalization by the girl, the reaction may be severe. Actions that seem justifiable on a moonlit evening with a date you like can look very sordid and stupid in the cold light of the next morning. In particular, a girl who has agreed to intercourse because she believed the boy was serious, and then finds that he doesn't care for her or isn't interested in continuing the relationship, frequently feels that she has betrayed herself. She may have persuaded herself that love made it right, and then finds that there was nothing but passing infatuation between them. In some cases she may persuade the boy into a disastrous marriage—or even convince herself that she is pregnant in order to procure a shotgun wedding which she hopes (mistakenly) will undo the wrong she feels she has done. Disgust and disillusion may make it difficult for her to establish confident, open communications with other boys. If you are going to be able to develop happy and satisfying sexual relationships it is important that your early experiences of intimacy be positive, warm, and free of guilt or resentment. If your first experience of intercourse is colored by disappointment or disillusion rather than by love and understanding, you start with a real disadvantage.

A girl who feels that her deepest emotions have been betrayed by a man, or that she has revealed her own unworthiness or instability, may drift into promiscuity. Here is the statement of one eighteen-year-old who had this experience: "Well, I'd meet boys, and get to know them— I'd *love* them, not just like them, so I stayed with them. . . . I didn't just go to anybody; I really liked those boys. But they used me. Like I'd tell them I liked them and wanted to be with them, and they'd use me and then say, 'Good-bye now, that's it.' And I was very hurt. . . . I think it was a good experience. I mean, I'm better now, I learned. I don't think everything I did was right, but I don't feel guilty. I mean it's just a misfortune that it went wrong. I learned about things and how to handle them. But even now I meet boys and the first thing they say is, 'Come on, let's go to bed.' And I want to show the boy that I like him, but now . . . I don't know what to do." The tragedy of this girl is that she hasn't really learned anything except that boys will take advantage of a girl who is free with her favors, and that once she acquires a reputation as an "easy lay" her chances of establishing deep relationships and regaining her self-esteem are slight.

What Is Virginity?

It has been said, with some truth, that it doesn't matter whether you are a virgn or not, but only *why* you are a virgin. Girls who avoid intercourse because they want to "save sex for marriage" may be merely masking a fundamental inability to relate to the other sex. Their reasons may be due to negative ideas about sex as something dirty, rather than to a responsible, honest decision to preserve the final intimacy of intercourse for the final commitment of marriage. One girl told me that she refused to sleep with her fiancé because she wanted to keep herself pure: but she had no objection whatever to his using other girls (for whom he had no affection at all) to satisfy his sexual needs. Other girls preserve a merely technical virginity by avoiding actual penetration, while allowing themselves to be petted to orgasm by a variety of boys. But to engage in such intimacy on a casual basis, without any real commitment, is surely more promiscuous than to go all the way with one boy you really love.

The *mere* preservation of an intact hymen, then, is not necessarily a mark of maturity or sexual integrity. But it remains true that the loss of virginity can have serious consequences for a girl in our society, which still stresses chastity as an ideal before marriage. Many boys still want to marry a girl who is a virgin, and regard a girl who sleeps with them as unfit for marriage. One boy put it like this: "I consider a girl you go out with and a girl you have intercourse with two different kinds of girls. There's a girl I date. I like to hold hands with her and make out with her, kiss her, but that's as far as I want to go with any girl I take out. If I like the girl I don't want to mess her up. But then, there is the other girls I just don't care about because they give it to the other guys—which means they don't care too much for theirselves."

But there is no point on which male attitudes are more contradictory: "Nobody would think of buying a pair of shoes without trying them on," goes the line, "so why should you expect me to marry you if you don't sleep with me first?" If the girl has any sense she'll point out that if he thinks of her as nothing more personal than a shoe he can't really love her. But if she goes along for the sake of preserving the relationship, the same boy may come to the conclusion that she's nothing but a tramp and show no further interest. Some boys quite consciously test a steady date or fiancée by trying to persuade her to go all the way, while secretly hoping she won't— and then reject her as "damaged goods" if she succumbs.

In some cases the loss of respect for the girl is merely a way of providing the boy with an excuse for his seduction or a reason for breaking off when the relationship is becoming more involved than he really wants. By persuading himself that the girl isn't, after all, respectable or reliable, he is able to clear his conscience of the guilt of seducing or abandoning her.

Boys Have Their Problems Too

While such attitudes show an appalling lack of sensitivity and little understanding of what love means, it would be quite inaccurate to suppose that boys are unaffected by the consequences of intercourse. We have to remember that the boy's natural biological urge toward intercourse is much stronger than that of the girl during the teens. He is encouraged by our culture to expect that intercourse will be infinitely more physically pleasurable than any other sexual experience, such as masturbation. The very fact that it is forbidden officially by adult society adds to the anticipation of special pleasure. But in practice the first attempt at intercourse often turns out to be far less thrilling than he expected. The earthquaking ecstasy proves to be a dud—though very few boys will admit this even to themselves, let alone to their friends. In the excitement he may ejaculate prematurely, penetration may be painful if the girl is a virgin or is not entirely relaxed, and even the achievement of orgasm is not by any means universal.

One of the reasons for failure, including incapacity to have an erection when it comes to the moment, may be that the boy is no more convinced than the girl that he really wants to engage in intercourse at this juncture. Group pressure, a desire to impress the girl, fears of inadequacy, response to adult teasing or challenges—any of these may temporarily override his basic moral and cultural convictions. At the critical point he may find it impossible to achieve orgasm, or he may do so mechanically but with a feeling of disgust and disillusionment. Religious objections he thought were dead and buried may prove stronger than instinct and lead to guilt which will adversely affect his future sexual development. Fears of parental discovery or disapproval may inhibit his free enjoyment of the experience. Two out of every five boys who have intercourse *even when they are engaged* report some feelings of guilt.

Further, most boys are aware, deep down, when they take advantage by protestations of love which are insincere, or pressures which make it difficult for the girl to say no. One boy when asked why he had not talked with his girl about having intercourse replied very honestly, "If you did that, you would talk yourself right out of it." Another boy gave this account of his experience: "I met a girl and started making love to her. Eventually she fell in love with me. (At least she thought she loved me and that, I think, amounts to the same thing. In other words, she could be badly hurt.) One day we were alone in my father's house and we decided to make love. This we accomplished in a bedroom on the second floor. After we finished, she wanted to be kissed and to hear that I loved her—anything at all that would *justify the act*. What she did not know was that *I felt nothing but a physical attraction* for her and wanted no part of her after we were finished. . . . For the first time I realized the damage I had done." For this boy who had the insight and humanity to see the truth, even after the event, such an experience was painful but probably beneficial. He had come to a new understanding of himself and of sex, which could lead to growth as a person and future happiness. But that could never undo the wrong he had done the girl and his memory of it.

The danger is, however, that some boys, rather than

gaining in sensitivity and responsibility as a result of early experiences of intercourse, may develop patterns of exploitative and superficial sexual behavior. Having discovered that you *can* persuade a girl to go all the way, and having enjoyed the physical satisfaction of intercourse, the temptation is to remain at this immature level of sexuality. The result may be that he grows up enjoying and using many sexual partners, but becomes incapable of establishing deep relationships with any single girl. Promiscuity is a symptom of basic personal inadequacy and insecurity; early habits of deceit and seduction may reinforce the underlying weakness of the individual and reduce his chances of healthy, stable development. A boy who succeeds in overcoming the hesitations of a girl may come to despise not only her but all women and may then find it impossible to enter into any trusting, healthy sexual union. Anyone who finds himself persisting in such activities should seek professional help before he develops patterns of behavior that are increasingly difficult to correct. Dr. Peter Bertocci addresses the following pertinent question to the boy who finds casual sexual intercourse enjoyable: "On what grounds does he expect to make an untroubled shift from sex-as-fun to sex as a means of expressing love in marriage? Does he expect the particular habits of emotional and bodily response which now regulate his sexual responsiveness to be easily transformed and to harmonize with the emotional and physical habits and expectations of his partner-in-love?"

The Alternative to Intercourse

Many boys, and an increasing number of girls, will rightly ask, "What is the alternative?" The steadily earlier onset of puberty and sexual desire, the increasing stimulation of erotic instincts by the media, the virtually unlimited freedom of social and sexual contact during adolescence, and the elimination of the traditional sanctions of pregnancy and VD—all of these seem to lead teenagers inevitably into intercourse. Boys need to develop their masculine self-identity in sexual encounters. Girls are anxious to discover whether they can measure up to the contemporary (and sometimes distorted) emphasis on orgasm as the test of feminine sexuality. Petting arouses sexual mechanisms which, if unsatisfied with release in orgasm, can lead to nervous tension, emotional frustration, and even to physical pain. Disappointment and irritation when sexual arousal is suddenly terminated short of climax can easily be transferred to the partner involved, so that negative rather than positive feelings result from what had been originally an expression of love and intimacy.

The solution increasingly accepted today is mutual petting to orgasm. Unfortunately, many adults (including some with otherwise enlightened attitudes to sexuality) still regard this practice as objectionable. It is not uncommon to hear it condemned as "mutual masturbation." But this description (which in any case assumes a wrongly negative view of masturbation) is quite unfair in many cases. Of course, heavy petting can be impersonal and purely physical, but some psychiatrists think that it is emotionally more suitable for young people. Petting to orgasm does allow many couples a profound intimacy, release from tension, and a means of maintaining their relationship until the final intimacy of intercourse can be enjoyed within the context of marriage.

It is clear from various studies that the distinction between heavy petting and actual intercourse is of particular importance to girls. Many girls report feelings of guilt and self-reproach following intercourse which they do not feel with any other type of sexual intimacy. For the boy intercourse is basically another experience of orgasm with the added pleasure which comes from the participation of the partner. For the girl intercourse involves a yielding of her inner being, a giving of her whole self, not merely an extension of the progression from kissing to petting. As one eighteen-year-old put it, "I like being kissed and cuddled, but I don't want them to sleep with me. I don't like the idea of someone else right inside me. Boys always want to go too far. They don't really pay you any attention, they just want your body." Any boy who claims seriously that "love makes it right" must therefore ask himself whether he should not deny himself the satisfaction of intercourse before marriage. Perhaps the argument should run: "Because I love her, I won't ask of her what she does not want to give" rather than "Because I love her, I have a right to what I want."

8 · Taking Care: Birth Control and Venereal Diseases

I said in the Introduction that I don't believe anyone can usefully lay down simple rules for you to regulate your sexual life by. But there are two principles that I believe any thinking person will accept as binding in all circumstances: "Do not conceive an unwanted child" and "Do not share VD." This chapter is intended to help you act in these ways as a responsible person.

The title of the chapter has two meanings. It is about what you need to do to take care about some possible results of intercourse. But equally importantly, it is about what it means to care for another person if you decide to go all the way. Nobody can seriously claim to love another if he or she does not take the necessary precautions to save the loved person from the risk of unwanted pregnancy or of disease. To call VD the "love bugs" is clever but entirely contradictory!

One very good argument against sexual intercourse in a casual, impersonal setting is that in those situations the risk of pregnancy is much higher. Some of the methods of birth control discussed in this chapter are very effective if they are properly used; but they are virtually useless if you don't apply them correctly. And using them effectively often depends on mutual caring between the couple. You will only avoid the risk of pregnancy if you are able to discuss the question openly in a context of trust and concern. You will be in serious danger of conceiving if you have intercourse when you are under pressure, embarrassed, hesitant, overwhelmed by passion or drugs or alcohol, swept away by romantic love, or acting on the spur of the moment because you're both sexually aroused.

Ineffective Methods of Birth Control

Teenagers often think quite wrongly that they can avoid pregnancy by the girl's not having an orgasm or by douching after intercourse. Whether the girl has an orgasm or not is *entirely* irrelevant to whether she gets pregnant. Douching is as likely to force sperm into the womb as it is to wash them out.

Two methods that can be quite helpful given certain conditions are not likely to work for teenagers. *Withdrawal* or "coitus interruptus," in which the boy's penis is withdrawn from the vagina before he ejaculates, calls for great skill and restraint on the part of the male, and even then doesn't guard against sperm that are discharged before ejaculation.

The *rhythm method* is the only form of birth control officially approved by the Catholic Church, although surveys indicate that a majority of Catholics do in fact make use of other means. The intention is to avoid pregnancy by having intercourse only on those days of each menstrual cycle when fertilization is impossible. For any individual woman in any particular month there are at most six days on which conception is possible, because of the limited life-span of ovum and sperm. However, variations in the date of ovulation in each cycle and variations in the length of each cycle for the same woman mean that in order to be safe, intercourse must be avoided for at least

eight days and by some for as many as sixteen days in
each month. The failure rate of the rhythm method is
twenty-four in every hundred women in a year—nearly
twice as many as the condom or the diaphragm, eight
times as many as the IUD, and eighty times as many as
the Pill. The chance of pregnancy can be reduced if the
woman is prepared to keep careful, regular records of
her temperature (which drops slightly at the time of ovulation) with a special thermometer. However this proce-
dure is thoroughly impracticable for teenagers. Even for
married couples it is objectionable to have to abstain from
intercourse for several days each month according to a
prescribed, mechanical timetable.

There is a "morning-after pill" which can be taken
after unprotected intercourse; but the chemical used
(DES) is very strong and carries serious risks to health.
You cannot get it from a doctor except in extreme
emergency.

Effective Methods of Birth Control

The contraceptives most used by teenagers are the condom and foam. Each by itself is quite effective—much
better than nothing—but used together (as they should
be) they are almost as reliable as the Pill. They have the
advantage that they can be bought at a drug store without
a prescription.

A *condom,* or "French letter" is a very thin synthetic
rubber sheath worn over the penis that prevents sperm
and semen from entering the vagina and, incidentally,
gives some protection against venereal disease. Modern
methods of manufacture pretty well ensure that each individual condom is reliable provided it is put on before
the penis comes into contact with the vagina.

Spermicidal foam is a white aerated cream containing a
sperm-killing chemical. It comes with a plastic applicator

with which the foam is placed in the vagina near the entrance to the cervix, thus preventing sperm from entering the uterus. Used by itself it is only fairly reliable, but if the boy also uses a condom the chances of conception are very slight. *Foam should not be confused with vaginal tablets or with "feminine hygiene products" such as Norforms, which are sometimes advertised as the solution to your "intimate marital problems."* These are not birth control methods at all and offer absolutely no protection.

The *Pill* is by far the most reliable means of birth control. There are in fact several types of pills, but they all work by modifying the female hormone balance so that no (ripe) eggs are released by the ovaries and therefore fertilization cannot take place. Their great advantage is that pregnancy occurs only three times in every *thousand* women in a year—a very small proportion. Their disadvantage is that absolute regularity in taking the Pill for a series of twenty-one days in each menstrual cycle is essential for full protection. Some women suffer side-effects such as weight increase or nausea, but these usually disappear after a few months' usage. Many million women in the United States have found the Pill entirely effective and safe. It does not either prevent or result in pregnancy when you cease to use it. The very slight risk of blood clots or other serious side effects is not likely to arise in young women, but it should be taken only under the direction of a qualified doctor or clinic and subject to regular checkups. It cannot be used by a girl who has not yet established a regular menstrual cycle.

Intrauterine devices (IUDs) are small plastic shapes that, when fitted in the uterus by a qualified person, prevent the egg from becoming attached to the wall of the womb so that it is expelled if it is fertilized. The advantage of the IUD is that, once inserted, it can remain in place for several years subject only to an annual checkup, and its operation does not depend upon human memory in taking a pill or counting the days of the month. Its disadvantage is that it can cause bleeding or cramps at first, and these sometimes continue, so that one woman out of three is unable to use an IUD. The proportion is somewhat higher among those who have not already had a pregnancy.

The *diaphragm* is a rubber cup inserted into the vagina so as to cover the neck of the womb and prevent sperm from entering. Used with a special spermicidal cream or jelly it is a very effective contraceptive. It must first be fitted by a medical professional and then inserted by the girl not more than six hours before intercourse.

Each couple must choose the method they are most comfortable with. It is important to avoid any method or device which you or your partner finds embarrassing or which interferes with sexual pleasure. Any method that is disturbing or found difficult to use is likely to be ineffective. Consciously or unconsciously there will be a tendency to forget to use it or to use it carelessly. And the result probably will be an unwanted pregnancy.

Venereal Diseases

It is estimated that some 80,000 people contract syphilis and two and a half million contract gonorrhea in the United States every year. Hundreds of thousands of these are teenagers, and the rate is increasing most rapidly in this age group.

Better health education and medical services have succeeded in stemming the increase of syphilis, but gonorrhea and herpes are virtually out of control and in epidemic proportions in every large American city.

Venereal diseases are no longer restricted to the poor and dirty, to the social outcast and to the urban centers. They are increasingly prevalent in rural and suburban communities, among professional and upper-class families. A promiscuous boy or girl will frequently pass on VD to dozens of people as the germs spread from one contact to another. Homosexual contacts are responsible for a good deal of syphilis. There is no way to be sure that any person who has had sexual contacts with a third party is free of infection.

You cannot get VD from dry toilet seats or towels, drinking fountains or dooknobs; but you do not have to have intercourse to become infected. Gonorrhea is almost always conveyed through the penis or the vagina, but syphilis can be caught through kissing, heavy petting, oral-genital sex, or anal contact, and herpes is spread through open sores on the genitals, thighs, or buttocks.

Syphilis is the most serious of the venereal diseases. Hundreds of people die of it every year in this country, and thousands more suffer physical and mental damage. The first sign is a hard, painless sore or ulcer (called a chancre) usually on the penis or near the vagina—sometimes on the mouth, tongue, or finger. This chancre appears a few weeks after infection, but it is easy to be misled by the fact that it disappears, *without* treatment, after two or three weeks. Thereafter the disease continues to spread, and the person continues to be infectious. However, diagnosis and cure are simple if treatment is sought in this period. Usually new symptoms occur a few months later: a rash (not always severe) on the hands or feet or the whole body, a sore throat, moist sores, or patches of baldness. These symptoms also eventually disappear though the disease continues. Even then, however, latent syphilis can be detected by a blood test and quickly halted by penicillin or some other antibiotic, though the damage already caused (often including the infection of the baby of a pregnant girl) cannot be reversed. Further delay will probably result in crippling disease or death.

Gonorrhea is seldom fatal but it is dangerous and (for

men in particular) very painful. It often causes sterility and crippling arthritis, sometimes serious damage to the heart. The first warnings for the male are a painful burning sensation when urinating and a thick milky discharge from the penis four days to a week after intercourse with an infected partner. Immediate treatment is essential if permanent damage is to be avoided. And while modern drugs are usually effective it is not simply a matter of a "couple of shots," since many strains of the germ gonococcus have become resistant to penicillin. Moreover, multiple infection with gonorrhea and syphilis is not uncommon, and reinfection is frequent.

Unfortunately, the treatment of gonorrhea in girls is much more difficult, and they have the additional risk of passing the disease on to any children they bear if they are not first rendered sterile. There is often no pain (though sometimes the female has the same burning sensation as the male when urinating) until serious harm has been done to the body. The milky discharge which men usually notice is slight and difficult for the girl to detect. Even a routine physical checkup is not likely to reveal the presence of gonorrhea, and a woman may carry and communicate the disease for years without knowing she has it.

Two other diseases which are often, though not always, spread by sexual intercourse have become common enough to require mention. *Herpes simplex* is a virus that causes painful blister-like sores on or near the genitals or anus. These soon heal but the disease remains latent and tends to erupt in times of stress. Women with herpes may be more liable to cervical cancer, may have difficulty carrying a fetus to full term, and may infect a baby at birth with serious consequences. *Venereal warts* are painless growths like hard, raised skin that appear usually on the vagina or penis several weeks after contact with an infected partner. They can be dealt with chemically or surgically.

If you have any reason whatsoever to think that you may have a venereal disease—either because of suspected symptoms or because you think you have had contact with someone who might have VD—it is essential to consult a physician or clinic. Remember to make it clear that you are worried about VD and not to ask merely for a general checkup. You may well have nothing more than acne, or a minor virus, but if treatment is needed it will be given sympathetically and confidentially. In the early stages recovery is usually simple, painless, and complete.

Many people fail to take the elementary precaution of seeking medical advice out of fear or shame. But today doctors and clinics are interested only in putting a stop to what are among the nation's most prevalent diseases. Professional people realize that the individual teenager is not especially to blame for the misfortune of contracting a sickness which is widespread among adults. Health authorities know that VD could be eliminated as completely as polio, but they need the cooperation of everyone. The only way the silent spread of disease can be stopped is by more accurate reporting of cases. If you have venereal disease the doctor is required to report the fact to the local health board, but *he will not usually tell your parents or anyone else unless you ask him to.* If you have reason to think your family doctor might break your confidence, go to someone who doesn't know you: he will not ask for any explanation. You will be asked to inform your contact and persuade him or her to get treatment.

9 · Teenage Marriage

The great playwright George Bernard Shaw is said to have been asked by a friend for advice about marriage, and to have replied on a postcard (as he often did) with the simple solution: "Don't!" Shaw's skepticism has not been widely shared, however; indeed, he didn't follow the advice himself. Nowadays a higher proportion of our population gets married than at any other time—and six out of seven people whose marriages fail try it again. Indeed, the high divorce figures, which are often quoted as evidence of the decline of the institution of marriage in our society may not reflect anything of the kind. Too easy divorce may tempt some people to treat their marriage vows lightly. But, while more liberal laws have made it easier for people to terminate the *legal* bonds of marriage, the number of marriages that break down (in the sense that the husband and wife no longer share any real sexual or emotional unity) may not have increased greatly. And while divorce is a sad experience for parents and children, it may be less tragic in the long run than the perpetuation of a merely formal marriage relationship when love and respect have died.

Many people seek divorce today because they have a higher, rather than a lower, idea of what marriage should mean. The emancipation of women has had the result of making modern marriage more a companionship of equals than an institution regulated by a legal contract. People are no longer satisfied to spend their lives sharing domestic arrangements without personal fulfillment or sexual satisfaction. Divorce or separation represent failure, but it is failure to achieve a goal to which other cultures and earlier generations have given little thought. The assumption that love and marriage *ought* to be related is almost unique to Western culture, and it's an ideal that's far from easy to achieve or to maintain.

Do Teenage Marriages Survive?

When it comes to marriage in the teens, the actual chances of achieveing worthwhile, strong marital-love relationships are greatly reduced. Students of contemporary problems in marriage and family life are virtually unanimous in echoing George Bernard Shaw's advice when it comes to teenage weddings: *Don't.* Failure in teenage marriage is about three times as likely as for the couple in their twenties—and there are 100,000 divorced or separated people in the United States today who are still in their teens. Of course, as we have said above, this may be the better of two evils—for a boy and girl who discover (usually within a year of the wedding day) that they are not really suited to each other, to be tied permanently would be even worse. But very few indeed of those who have been through the experience of early marriage and divorce recommend it to others. The disappointment and bitterness leave emotional scars that are often serious and permanent. Relationships are established that can never be totally erased. Experiences and hopes are spoiled so that they cannot be shared with the same freshness in a second marriage. And second marriages more often end in divorce than first marriages.

The basic reason for failure in teenage marriages is the very simple and obvious one—at that stage of life many of us are not yet sufficiently clear in our understanding of our own characters or of the qualities we really want in a life partner. To choose a wife or a husband is to make a decision about your future personal and social development. It will affect your friendships and family ties, the kind of children you have, and the atmosphere of the home you live in. It may ultimately enrich or stifle your personal abilities, your capacity for creative contributions to society, or your prospects in a career or profession. It may make all the difference in the world between emotional happiness or breakdown, between terrible loneliness or inspiring comfort in sickness or financial hardship. Every marriage contains a large element of uncertainty—not only because none of us fully understands himself or herself, but also because the experience of marriage produces changes in the personalities of both partners. Teenagers, moreover, are much more likely than people in their twenties or thirties to undergo radical modifications of character; and if this happens during the crucial first years of marriage, the strains of marital adjustment are very greatly increased. Demands of patience, and sensitivity which might be met in the context of later life all too often prove excessive when the confusions and misunderstandings of adolescent self-development must also be taken into account.

Infatuation Or Love?

Because sex and love are so new and wonderful in adolescence, teenagers are more likely than older couples to marry on the basis of mere infatuation. There is a widespread tendency in the first flush of exhilaration and joy to ignore all the facts and fall back into totally unrealistic assumptions about romantic love. Despite the experience of others—often of one's own friends—entirely false notions are allowed to befog the mind and exclude rational discussion. Such potentially disastrous misunderstandings as the following are not uncommon: "When you fall head-over-heels in love, it's sure to be the real thing." "It doesn't matter if you don't know your partner well, or share common interests, provided you're truly in love." "Love at first sight is usually the deepest and most enduring kind." "There's only one ideal mate for each person, and you know instinctively if you've found him (or her), so there's no point in discussing it with other people." What happens here is that some truth—"You just know when you're really in love"; "love can't be objectively studied"; "love is important as a basis for marriage," etc.—is erroneously taken to imply an obvious falsehood—obvious, that is, except to the befuddled individual who makes the statement. For, as a matter of sheer fact, hundreds of thousands of people who have married because they were hopelessly, dramatically, and rapturously in love have found out within a year or so that the person they married was not right for them. On the other hand, hundreds of thousands of people who have *not* married the boy or girl they were first (or second or third) in love with have met and happily married another boy or girl later on.

The basic ingredient in romantic self-delusion is, of course, the natural sexual instinct. But sociological and psychological factors can play a significant part in persuading the teenager that a particular girl or boy is the final answer to his or her dreams. A girl who is tired of the uncertainty and demands of the dating game may be tempted to find an easy solution to fears of spinsterhood by idealizing a very ordinary and quite inappropriate boy who wants her as a wife. A couple who are under pressure from their friends to tie the knot because "they're obviously meant for each other" can all too easily capitulate because it's the easy way out. They may not really be suited, or even deeply in love, but merely conforming to group expectations. Marriage in other cases may be used as a means of achieving adult stat_s and freedom, and the boy or girl who has previously been denied the privileges of adulthood is likely to be least prepared for the responsibilities and demands of early married life.

Parental Pressures

The quality of our relationships to our parents can be even more important in affecting our judgment about marriage. An adolescent who has not been able adequately to establish his identity as a person before he falls in love is very liable to transfer his childhood dependence directly to the girl. She seems to him to satisfy all his needs as a potential wife, but fundamentally he is attracted to her as a substitute mother. Since like often attracts like, she may make the same mistake, with the result that they find soon after marriage that neither is strong or mature enough to meet the demands of the other. On the other hand, many teenage marriages which involve cross-racial, cross-class, or interfaith unions are basically disguised expressions of rebellion rather than profound love relationships. Marriages that cut across traditional social or cultural boundaries can and do succeed. But if the unconscious motive that attracts two people from different backgrounds is their need to confound parental expectations, they will probably find that once they have hoisted the flag of independence, they have insufficient emotional resources to sustain them in their isolation against the additional strains of a socially unconventional marriage. If you marry young *because* your parents think you should wait, you may be successful in showing them who's running your life; but you may not have enough real commitment to your partner in freedom to maintain the marriage till you're much older.

When Marriage Is A Crutch

Problems of this kind are not, of course, the fault of the couple involved. As we have seen in earlier chapters, the personality is formed by the interaction of the individual and the subtle forces of family, peer group, and society at large—though in a mysterious way the individual acquires some responsibility for what he is and does. That is what it means to be a person and not merely a battleground of warring instincts. Marriage, when it is based on real love and honest self-understanding, can help people to develop their strengths and rise above some of their weaknesses. But if marriage is entered into primarily as a therapeutic measure, as a means to solve serious personality problems, it seldom delivers what is wanted. This danger is present, of course, in marriage at any age but there is a special temptation for the teenager to use marriage as a crutch to carry the weight of personal weakness. It is all too easy to treat the beloved unconsciously as a nurse or doctor equipped with a magical nostrum to heal your inner sickness. Instead of working out the various stages of adolescence through continuing confrontation and communication with a variety of people (including, of course, members of the other sex), the individual retreats into early marriage only to find that no one else can solve his or her problems. All too often the very same inadequacies in family relationships that have adversely affected a person's growth are merely reproduced in the new family unit. In some cases later marriage would be no more successful; but in many others delay might allow the individual to develop greater integrity and strength before facing the additional challenges of early marital adjustment.

What About Trial Marriage?

In view of the difficulties involved in making a responsible and reliable choice of a marriage partner for life, it is not surprising that many people have raised the possibility of radical changes in our pattern of marriage. "If there is so much danger of a wrong decision about a permanent union," it is asked, "why not modify the basic intention of marriage and accept the fact that a young couple are only ready for a temporary arrangement? Why not allow them, with the approval of society, to live together for a trial period? Then, if they find they are well matched, the marriage can be continued; but if serious problems arise it can be terminated without undue pain or embarrassment."

There is something to be said for people living together before marriage in order to get to know each other as fully as possible. It is, of course, much more common today and we can only hope that those who try the experiment will make wiser choices of a marriage partner than in the past. But there is a fundamental difference between a marriage that allows in advance for escape if the going gets rough and one that is undertaken (at least in principle) for life. In any preliminary or trial arrangement the couple is trying each other out rather than living together in a commitment. Marriage, on the other hand, is essentially not an opportunity to test the other person's qualities *before* deciding to share your life, your goods, your body, and your future: it is the experience of actually sharing these things. However risky it may be, the decision to share them with this particular partner through sickness and health is integral to the nature of the project. You cannot really have a trial marriage any more than you can have a trial pregnancy.

Marriage specialists generally agree that without the assumption that marriage is for keeps, many more couples would fail in the demanding but worthwhile task of building a successful relationship. As the anthropologist Margaret Mead concluded: "No known society has ever invented a form of marriage strong enough to stick that did not contain the 'till-death-do-us-part' assumption." The fact that the union is final, not subject to review if it proves demanding, is a major factor in stabilizing the situation during a crisis and helping a husband and wife to persist in adaptation and growth. Most happily married people will agree that they have only really understood what love can mean when they have survived together the kind of strain that would soon bring any less permanent relationship to an end. If you are free to terminate the bond between you when it is in danger of disintegrating, you will probably never know what it means to achieve your real potential of love (including sexual satisfaction). The paradox of marriage is that you can't really discover its depths and joys without committing yourself fully to one man or one woman; but you can't be sure he or she is the one to whom you should be committed until you're well and truly involved in the give-and-take of marriage—and probably of parenthood.

Does Formal Engagement Help?

On the whole, therefore, it seems more profitable to give attention to the problems involved in the choice of a partner than to ways of making that choice less decisive. So we shall conclude this book with some suggestions about mate selection. For while I started this chapter by saying that the first piece of advice to teenagers contemplating marriage should be "Don't," it would be a great mistake to make that the last word. Unfortunately, adults tend to be suspicious of all teenage marriages and to assume that the girl is pregnant or the couple hopelessly impulsive. All too often one of these fears is justified. But many boys and girls are mature enough for marriage in their teens and many early marriages prove to be wonderful and lasting experiences. Given the understanding and support of their families, a couple who are mature and in love may sometimes be well advised *not* to wait. But only those who are able and ready to take a good long look at each other and achieve some objectivity in their relationship should take this step. There is certainly no need to puncture all the idealizations of love (few of us would even take the step of marriage if we did that); but the camouflage of romantic role-play must be lifted so that honest encounter is possible.

Formal engagement has its advantages and its disadvantages. It indicates that a couple expect to get married and makes it possible for them to turn from the preliminaries of attracting each other to the serious business of considering whether their love is strong enough to sustain them for life. Studies indicate that long engagements are favorable to marital success: they should not last less than six months; a full year is better. On the other hand, a formal engagement can become burdensome if it is forgotten that engagements are made to be broken, if the couple find that they are not after all capable of surviving the mutual self-testing involved. If, out of a mistaken sense of pride or loyalty or embarrassment, engagement leads to the hiding of facts and attitudes which might undermine the relationship, it fails entirely to fulfill its function. What is needed is that the boy and girl spend as much time as possible in nonsexual situations observing, examining, and criticizing each other. If the prospects of healthy marriage are to be increased, the period of engagement will involve a good deal of disillusionment, some serious disagreements, and the growth of unselfish love which can accept the partner's limitations without losing faith in his or her essential value.

Some Questions To Ask

The kind of questions that have to be raised are these: Has he a reasonable record for reliability in school or work? Is she able to make up her own mind without referring every issue to mother? Does he take her for granted now that she's agreed to marriage? Can she cope with the daily chores of household management and keep to a budget? Does one of you unconsciously despise the other for reason of color or religion? What do people who know him best think about his qualities as a husband? Do her parents seem aware of her weaknesses or do they always try to sell her as a perfect wife? Does he react violently to criticism or disagreement? Does she respond negatively whenever you propose a change from routine? Do you differ radically in your ideas about bringing up children? Does he (or she) show signs of being a hypochondriac? Are either of you basically envious of the other's educational achievements or class background? Does he expect the woman in his life to act as a personal maid, polishing his shoes and cleaning up after his bath? Does she put on a front when out on dates but drop into slovenly habits at home? Failure to measure up to ideal standards on every count need not result in breaking the engagement, but it is unrealistic to suppose that your prospective husband or wife is going to change dramatically during the wedding ceremony. You may have reasonable hopes of modifying minor traits over the years, but the question is whether you can live with your partner's real self, warts and all, long enough to make any impression.

It's not necessary for a happy marriage that a husband and wife agree on everything. Indeed, domestic life would be very dull if this were the case. But there may be some things about which they disagree so strongly that they lack the patience and love to transcend the difference. And it is important that each of them should be aware of the other's point of view on matters of controversy before they have to be faced within marriage. Issues about which they could have agreed to differ may become serious irritants if an unsuspected divergence of opinion comes into the open only after marriage has been entered into. Disappointment, disillusion, and even suspicion may aggravate the problem if the partner's views on politics, race, or religion have been taken for granted and then turn out to be radically contrary to one's own. Here are some basic questions that must be discussed in advance:

How do you view the respective roles of husband and wife?   Which of you is to be responsible for overall budgeting or (as most experts would advise) are you going to share financial responsibilities? Is the husband going to participate in household chores? Is the wife going to continue her education or drop out of school? Will she go to work, and if she does will she be free to spend her salary independently?

How do you feel about your in-laws?   If your fiancé or fiancée refuses to take you home to meet your prospective in-laws, for whatever apparently good reason, look out for trouble. It may be justifiable, but it may be that you are being used, unconsciously, as a means of escape from an intolerable situation—or that your future husband or wife is secretly ashamed or jealous of you. Several *long* visits together with each set of parents are desirable, particularly if your marriage is to cross racial, religious, or cultural boundaries. Only in this way can you assess your future spouse's relationship to the mother and father—a relationship which is bound to affect his or her attitude as husband or wife and parent.

Inevitably one has a special bond with one's own parents, and it is natural to defend them and depend on them in a crisis; but a truly healthy relationship should make it possible for a couple contemplating marriage to be objective between themselves about parental oddities. Each should be able to talk honestly about in-laws and the role they will play in the marriage. And if either the boy or the girl shows a tendency to run back to mother when things get difficult, it is doubtful that he or she is really ready for an independent existence in a new family unit.

How much of your free time will you spend together? Some marriages are shipwrecked in the first few months because the young wife finds that her husband takes it for granted he can go out with the boys whenever he wants, and no longer bothers to entertain her. Or a husband may complain that his wife's time is so taken up with church activities she has no time to talk with him in the evenings. It's a good thing to have some interests ouside the family circle, but in marriage you have to learn new patterns of recreation. The fact that one of the two doesn't care for television or classical music or skiing may not matter when you're dating or engaged—each of you has other things to attend to. But unless you're prepared for it, life in an apartment can be very tense or very lonely if your mate spends a lot of time in some relaxation you can't share—tense if it's something like pop tunes on the stereo or cards with the neighbors, lonely if it's coaching the Little League or taking evening classes in drawing. And remember that a boy or a girl who participates in the teenage social scene because it's the only way to meet people may be looking forward eagerly to getting married and enjoying quiet evenings by the (metaphorical) fireside. If he or she picks a partner who's enthusiastic about socializing the result can be disappointment and marital failure.

What are your expectations about sex in marriage? Despite the impression given by the marriage manuals, complete mutual sexual satisfaction is by no means easy or automatic in the early months of marriage, and serious problems can arise if either of the partners has expectations that are unfulfilled. The first thing to be emphasized is that any difficulties encountered are likely to be due to emotional factors which can be corrected with understanding and patience, and *not* to any physical inadequacy or permanent psychological disorder. Many teenagers imagine that difference in the size of the male and female genital organs is a source of maladjustment, but this is virtually never the case. Very occasionally the girl's hymen is unusually tough and needs treatment by a minor surgical incision. If penetration proves impossible or very painful after several attempts at intercourse, a doctor should be consulted. But otherwise the vagina is remarkably adaptable, and both partners can obtain full satisfaction however large or small the male penis may be.

The idea that it is important to have intercourse before marriage in order to find if the couple are suited physically is therefore nonsense. In many cases the achievement of sexual fulfillment depends on having the opportunity to engage in intercourse in the secure, unhurried, confident context of marriage. If a couple try to test out their physical compatibility in circumstances of fear and discomfort before the decisive commitment of marriage has been made, the result may be entirely misleading. Because one or the other of them is anxious about discovery or pregnancy, or has religious and ethical reservations, they may be unsuccessful. If they then conclude that they are unable to "fit down there," a relationship which is basically sound may be terminated because of entirely temporary factors which could be readily overcome after marriage.

Complex emotional forces can affect sexual performance. A man may ejaculate prematurely because of anxiety about his sexual prowess or the excitement of participating in intercourse for the first few times. A woman, particularly if she has been the subject of embarrassing or disappointing sexual experiences in earlier life, may have difficulty in relaxing sufficiently to allow full penetration. Patience, tact, encouragement, and above all accurate knowledge are vital if progress is to be made and frustration avoided. It may be advisable for the husband to have an orgasm through petting first, and then a little later to proceed to intercourse. The wife will almost certainly need to be reassured and aroused by expressions of love, petting, and foreplay, including the manual stimulation of the clitoral area. If her husband withdraws immediately after his climax and goes to sleep without helping her to reach orgasm, she may be left frustrated and dissatisfied. If either partner approaches intercourse with selfish impatience or makes no effort to respond sensitively to the needs of the other, failure is inevitable.

It cannot be sufficiently stressed that success in early marital sex does *not* depend upon the wife being able to have an orgasm actually during intercourse—through the stimulation of the clitoris by the man's penis. We now know that many women never have an orgasm during intercourse, and many more do not do so until they have been married for some years or perhaps until they have had a child. This is not to say they do not want or need the pleasure of orgasm; but they may depend on extensive petting by their partner or, if he is unconcerned, on masturbation to reach satisfaction.

A great deal of unnecessary distress results from the

mistaken assumption that all women can readily climax
during intercourse. Wives who fail to enjoy this expecta-
tion on the wedding night may quite wrongly conclude
that they are lacking in sexuality. A husband who assumes that his wife will automatically "come" when he
does may be plagued by fears that he is lacking in masculinity, or even worse he may begin to suspect or accuse
her of "frigidity." Psychiatrists report a growing incidence
of "pseudo-frigidity" in which young wives are incapable
of enjoying intercourse because their husbands have ac-
cused them of being frigid or perverted if they need
manual stimulation to achieve orgasm. Thus a tragic vi-
cious circle of recrimination, self-contempt, anxiety, and
increased difficulty in sexual response results. Because
more is expected than some women either need or want,
unjustified disappointment can wreck a potentially happy
marriage.

Sexual Satisfaction in Marriage

The essential ingredient for sexual fulfillment is mutual
concern, so that sex becomes not a matter of personal
prowess or the satisfaction of individual physical needs,
but the expression of self-giving love in the unity of two
selves. It can become not less but more pleasurable and
satisfying as the couple grow in sensitivity to each other's
physical needs. But this will not happen by accident.
Some men give up love-making once they have acquired
the "rights" of a husband. Some wives think it no longer
necessary to make themselves attractive once they have
got their man. A husband has to learn when his wife's
sexual desires are highest (probably just after or before
her period). A wife has to learn that a man may be less
erotically inclined when he's depressed by his work. Each
has to learn not to take these temporary changes in sexual enthusiasm as if they reflected any lessening of love

for the partner. On the other hand, in early married life
a woman may have to satisfy her husband's urgent needs
for relief when she would prefer to drop off to sleep, and
in later years a husband may have to initiate love-making
when he would personally just as well pass it up. In
happy sexual adjustment there is no rule to say intercourse must take place so many times a week, any more
than there is any physical rule that says it shouldn't take
place so many times a night. Sexual fulfillment is reached
when a couple can sense and respond to each other's love
without reservation, embarrassment, or pressure—and
that takes a lot of consideration, patience, and frank discussion. Young people tend to think that sexual passion
ceases as you approach thirty. But a Roper poll found
that married people reported *increased* sexual satisfaction
in one out of four instances, equal satisfaction with the
early years of marriage in one out of three cases, and a
decline in sexual pleasure in only one out of four marriages.

One further aspect of sexual adjustment that can cause
trouble is the question of what is "natural" or "normal" in
sex. Nowadays most psychiatrists and many religious
teachers recognize that any type of sexual intimacy between married couples, provided it is mutually desired
and expressive of affection, is entirely harmless unless it
becomes an obsessive substitute for intercourse. But the
important qualification is "mutually desired." If one
partner is privately embarrassed or disgusted with some
practice the other wishes to engage in, the seeds of resentment may be sown. If the wife or husband dislikes
some positions for intercourse, shares the old-fashioned
taboo against intercourse during menstruation or early
pregnancy, or finds oral-genital contact repellent, nothing but unhappiness will come from the attempt to override such hesitations. In many cases they will disappear
with time and increasing trust or knowledge.

The Question of Children

Perhaps the most vital question for teenagers contemplating marriage is *What are your plans about parenthood?* In many cases, of course, teenage marriages are contracted because the girl is already pregnant. Marriage seems an obvious solution to the problem of an unwanted baby. But despite the fact that adults are likely to exert great pressure on teenagers to take this way out, the demand should be resisted. A "shot-gun" wedding has some advantages for the parents of the couple (particularly of the girl), because it saves them the embarrassment of illegitimacy in the family. It may temporarily relieve the guilt felt by the boy and girl themselves. But in the long run the advantages are likely to be greatly outweighed by disadvantages for the couple and for the child.

Pregnancy is undoubtedly among the major factors leading to early teenage divorce. Because they start their married life with immediate financial burdens and additional demands on their time and energy, the vital task of adjusting to marriage and learning to live together is greatly complicated. Both partners feel restricted in their opportunities of social contact with their friends, and the mother in particular finds herself tied night and day to the care of an infant she does not really want. Each is liable (perhaps silently) to blame the other for the predicament, thus raising barriers to understanding and love between them. Worst of all (again usually unconsciously but even more deeply) both are liable to blame the baby for their troubles. The widespread idea that marriage is best for the sake of the unborn child is very questionable. A baby adopted by people who want a child and cannot have their own, or even a baby brought up by its mother alone, is much more likely to develop a happy, strong personality than a child who discovers that its parents resent it for having tied them unwillingly together.

If a couple is really in love and has the personal maturity to overcome the additional strains of early parenthood a very different situation exists, and many marriages have developed into strong and wonderful relationships following premarital pregnancy. However, even if a couple is deeply commmitted and pregnancy results from a long period of engagement, it is best not to be impelled into marriage unless you are quite sure you want each other for life. Some people who were very much in love before pregnancy find that the crisis shows up basic suspicions, distrust, unreadiness for permanent commitment, or immaturities of some other kind that were unsuspected before. It is interesting that in Sweden, where the unmarried mother and illegitimate baby are far less subject to social embarrassment than in this country, a considerable proportion of couples who have been engaged decide not to be married once pregnancy occurs. This suggests that many couples find that becoming responsible for the conception of a baby does not cement their relationship but destroys it, and that where they are free from public pressure, they prefer to separate. It's difficult to face these facts, especially when friends and parents are likely to ignore them; but it's better to be honest and part company than to gloss over deep gulfs and enter on marriage lacking the essential resources of mutual confidence and trust.

In most cases the avoidance of pregnancy is equally desirable within the first year or two of a teenage marriage. Time is needed for the couple to discover each other fully and to establish solid foundations of personal and sexual unity before they have to face the additional strains and financial burdens of parenthood. The privileges and joys of loving and caring for children can be a tremendous strength to a marital relationship when the parents are ready for this role. But if a baby comes too soon, one or both of them may be denied the opportunity to complete his or her education or professional training, with the result that the unfortunate child can become the object of unconscious resentment and strife. All too many unwanted pregnancies originate during the honeymoon because it is mistakenly assumed that the risks are worth taking until a doctor can be consulted. In fact the chances of conceiving during the exciting and often intense sexual activity of the first few weeks are quite high. Every engaged couple should consult a doctor before the marriage to discuss methods of contraception and to have a thorough medical checkup.

One subject about which honest discussion before marriage is important is the controversial issue of abortion. Now that abortion is legal in the United States it is inevitable and proper that a couple consider it if an unwanted pregnancy occurs. When performed in a reputable clinic *up to the* twelfth week after the girl's last menstrual period, it is a safe and relatively simple operation and does not require overnight stay. There is no real evidence to support the view that abortion generally results in severe depression or permanent psychological damage. In many cases the strains of bringing up an unwanted baby are likely to be more serious. A girl who has other emotional problems may find that these are brought to a head by the experience of abortion; but the same is likely to be true if she has to look after a baby she does not want.

The decision to terminate pregnancy cannot be lightly made. Many people have profound religious or moral objections to abortion, and every couple has to take these factors into account in making a decision whether to seek abortion if an unwanted pregnancy has occurred. Anyone who believes that the fetus is a human being with a soul from the moment of conception, and that abortion (unless it occurs indirectly as a result of efforts to save the life of the mother) is equivalent to murder is likely to suffer severe guilt feelings if she has an abortion. On the other hand, if each is able to accept abortion, it may save the marriage from intolerable strains in the early years, and enable them to be much better parents to a wanted child later on.

Love in Marriage

In conclusion, if you hope to achieve long-standing happiness in marriage you need to face the question: *What do you expect of love?*

There is a tendency for teenagers to fear (with reason when they contemplate some of the marriages they observe around them) that love dies when a relationship is given formal expression in marriage. To some extent as the novelty wears off (maybe that's a good reason for not trying everything before you're eighteen!), the intensity and excitement of love and sex decline. But you will bemoan this only if you have false expectations based on a one-sided identification of love and romanticism. If you expect to feel the same thrill every time you see your wife or husband at breakfast after ten years as you do now when you meet for an hour or two several times a week, you're just plain stupid. If you think that losing that effervescent, spine-tingling feeling means the end of love, you're bound for a disappointment. Mere age will take care of that: like it or not, the metabolism of the human body changes and the man or woman in the twenties or thirties just can't react the way he (or she) did at fifteen or eighteen. Heaven forbid that married love should lose its spontaneity altogether. A marriage in which the man never catches his breath when he sees his wife undress, or the woman's heartbeat never quickens at her husband's touch is in trouble. But a relationship which consisted of nothing more than romance would be as unsubstantial and as heady as a continuous diet of the champagne you may drink (if you're lucky) at your wedding.

Erma Bombeck in a column in the *Cleveland Plain Dealer** headed "Love . . . Poets Don't Tell It Like It Is" made the point better than I can:

An English assignment by my daughter the other night wrung a confession out of me which is almost un-American. "Elizabeth Barrett Browning always made me a little sick to my stomach," I said. "She reminded me of a politician's wife standing at her husband's elbow grinning adoringly like she had horse feathers in her underwear. I only said I liked her so my English teacher would think I was a sensitive girl."

"Don't you think it was romantic the way she wrote, 'How do I love thee? Let me count the ways'?"

"That isn't love," I said. "That's worship. Love is a lot of little things that are basic."

"Like what?" she countered.

"Well, you love a man who can teach you how to drive the car without giving you a karate chop for stripping the gears. Or a man who proposes so awkwardly he says, 'Do you wanta get married . . . or what?' Or a husband who doesn't tell his mother how he broke his tooth eating your white sauce.

"You love a man who doesn't faint, leave town or hang one on when you tell him you're going to have a baby. Or a thoughtful man who won't drink coffee or fry bacon in the house during your first three months.

"You love a man who will take out the garbage even though he's a college graduate. Or a man who isn't ashamed to wash a dish or change a diaper.

"You love a man who will stick by you when you have the mumps at 24, or says you're beautiful when you have a tooth pulled.

"You love a man who laughs at your joke—every time you tell it—and a man who smiles at your mother.

"You love a man who says his old girl friend looks

* June 20, 1968. Reprinted with permission.

frumpy. Who doesn't wait until Christmas Eve to put up a
Christmas tree. Who doesn't talk about money during din-
ner. Who lies about his vacation with the 'boys' and says
he's glad to be home. Who says at least once a year, 'You
want to dance?'

"You love a man who brings you a box of punch-and-
grow tomato seeds when it wasn't even on the grocery list.
A man who has the decency not to laugh about your 40th
birthday. A man who knows when to be amorous, when to
keep silent, when to smile, when to be on time, when to be
late, when to get his wife out of the house before she falls
out of her tree."

Love is something you have to cultivate and learn, with
humility, courage, faith, and discipline. That, after all, is
the real reason why most people get married in church or
synagogue. The religious service is not a legal formality,
it is an acknowledgment that none of us can hope to fulfill all the responsibilities and possibilities of love and sex
without help. A wedding is more than a public acknowledgment of our commitment—though that is important:
it is also a means of grace, a symbol or a sacrament
through which you hope to receive God's help in building
a healthy marriage. If you expect of love that the thrill of
romance and pleasure in each other will carry you
through life without effort, you are riding for a fall. But
if you expect of love that it will demand care and concern, pain and tears, you may just discover how profoundly wonderful marriage can be. The romance of adolescence will not be lost but fulfilled in a lasting union of
love. The intensity of teenage joy will find its natural fru-
ition in mature adult relationship. If you grow up with sex
as a joyful privilege rather than a selfish lust or an anxious burden, you will be a *whole* person.

What the Sex Words Mean

Abortion: The expulsion of the embryo or fetus from the womb before it is capable of independent life. An accidental or spontaneous abortion is usually called a **Miscarriage.**

Adolescence: The period between puberty and adulthood.

Adultery: Sexual intercourse between two people, one or both of whom are married to another person. In most states adultery is against the law.

Anus (Anal): The opening through which the body's solid waste matter is discharged from the bowel.

Aphrodisiac: A drug intended to arouse sexual desire. From the Greek title for the goddess of love. Those (very few) aphrodisiacs which are effective are dangerous; those which are harmless are almost entirely useless.

Bisexual: Someone who engages in sexual activity with members of either sex.

Brothel: A house where prostitutes are available. From the Old English word meaning "a ruined, abandoned person."

Climax: See **Orgasm.**

Conception: The uniting of sperm and ovum to initiate a new life.

Contraceptive: Any device that prevents conception or fertilization.

Contraceptive Jelly: A chemical substance used in connection with contraceptive devices such as the diaphragm, which kills sperm and thus helps to reduce the risk of fertilization.

Copulate: To have sexual intercourse. From the Latin word meaning "couple" or "join together."

Cunnilingus: Oral stimulation of the female genitals.

Deviant: Differing from what is normal or conventional.

Diaphragm: A rubber contraceptive cup inserted in the vagina so as to cover the neck of the womb and prevent sperm from entering.

Don Juan: A man who seeks sexual conquests purely to demonstrate his virility or prowess. Derived from the reputation of a fourteenth century Spaniard later immortalized in literature.

Douche: An instrument which directs a stream of water into the vagina. Sometimes used (ineffectively) as a contraceptive.

Ejaculation: The expulsion of sperm and semen from the penis at the climax of sexual stimulation.

Ejaculatio Praecox: See **Premature Ejaculation.**

Embryo: The growing baby in the mother's womb, from the time the zygote attaches itself to the womb wall until the body parts can be distinguished at about three months (when it is called the fetus).

Epididymis: The network of tubes behind and above the testicles in which sperm are stored.

Erection: The stiffening and enlargement of the penis, due to increased flow of blood, which makes possible insertion into the vagina during intercourse.

Erogenous Zones: Those parts of the body most sensitive to sexual arousal—the genitals, female breasts, mouth etc. From the Greek word for love.

Erotic: Pertaining to physical sexual desire. From the Greek word for love, which originally referred also to love of truth, beauty, etc.

Exhibitionism: A condition in which the person—usually a man—feels a need to expose his genitals publicly or to make obscene telephone calls to women.

Fallopian Tubes: The ducts which convey the ovum from the ovary to the uterus, and in which conception takes place. Named after their discoverer, a sixteenth-century anatomist.

Fellatio: Oral stimulation of the male genitals.

Fertile: Capable of growing into or producing a living thing.

Fertilization: The union of a male sperm and female ovum in the Fallopian tube, producing a new life or zygote.

Fetus: The growing baby in the mother's womb after the embryo has developed distinct body parts, at about three months.

Foam: A sperm-killing substance inserted into the vagina as a means of birth control.

Foreplay: Kissing, hugging and caressing by which a couple stimulate each other in preparation for intercourse.

Foreskin: The covering of the tip or glans of the penis, which is removed in many cases (by circumcision) soon after a boy is born.

Fornication: Sexual intercourse between two unmarried persons. Illegal in many states. The word comes from the Bible, where it normally refers to sexual acts of a purely impersonal and promiscuous kind.

Freud, Sigmund: The father of modern psychiatry (1856–1939) whose ideas, while not accepted uncritically, have profoundly illuminated our understanding of sexuality.

Frigidity: Disinterest in (but not necessarily incapacity for) sexual experience. Normally applied to women. From the Latin for "cold." Usually, but not always, due to psychological rather than physical causes, and dependent on varying circumstances.

Genitals: The external sex organs, male or female. From the Latin word meaning "to beget or conceive."

Glans: The tip of the penis, reddish-purple in color.

Gonads: The sex glands—ovaries in the female, testicles in the male.

Gonorrhea: The most widespread venereal disease, almost always contracted by sexual intercourse.

Hermaphrodite: An (extremely rare) individual who possesses the sex glands (testicles and ovaries) of both sexes. Originally the name of the (mythical) offspring of the Greek god Hermes and the goddess of love Aphrodite.

Herpes Simplex: A viral disease, one form of which is apparently spread by sexual contact.

Heterosexual: A person whose sexual desire is directed in adulthood towards members of the other sex.

Homosexual: A person who prefers in adulthood to achieve sexual satisfaction with a member of the same sex. From the Greek word meaning "same," *not* from the Latin for "man." See **Lesbian.**

Hormone: A chemical substance which affects the growth of the body. The primary male sex hormone (androgen) and the primary female sex hormones (estrogen and progesterone) control the growth of secondary sexual characteristics such as breasts, hair, etc.

Hymen: A thin membrane almost covering the entrance of the vagina in most (but not all) girls before they have engaged in intercourse.

Impotence: Inability of the male to achieve and maintain erection and have intercourse. Usually, but not always psychological in origin. From the Latin for "loss of power."

Incest: Sexual relations between close relatives.

Infertility: The condition of being unable to produce offspring. Due usually to lack of sufficient live sperm or ova, sometimes to inability of the sperm to reach the female egg. Often capable of cure under medical supervision. See **Sterility.**

Intercourse: The insertion of the penis into the vagina.

Intrauterine Device (IUD): A contraceptive which is inserted by a doctor and prevents the attachment of the fertilized egg to the wall of the uterus.

Kinsey, Alfred Charles: The primary author of the famous reports *Sexual Behavior in the Human Male* (1948) and *Sexual Behavior in the Human Female* (1953).

Labia Majora: The outer fold of the female external genitals or vulva. Literally "the greater lips" (Latin).

Labia Minora: The inner fold of the female external genitals or vulva. Literally "the lesser lips" (Latin).

Lesbian: A female homosexual. From the name of the Greek island (Lesbos) where the poetess Sappho (600 B.C.), who was thought to be homosexual, lived.

Libido: Freud's word for the basic sexual drive. Derived (most unfortunately) from the Latin for "lust."

Masochism: A condition in which the individual derives sexual pleasure only through being subjected to humiliation or pain. From the name of a nineteenth century author who wrote about people suffering from this disorder.

Masters & Johnson: Dr. William H. Masters and Mrs. Virginia E. Johnson, authors of *Human Sexual Response* (1966) and *Human Sexual Inadequacy* (1970), two important studies of the physical aspects of sexual activity.

Masturbation: The self-stimulation of the genitals (male or female) by the hands or other means to achieve orgasm. Probably meaning "hand-defilement."

Menopause: The "cessation of menses" or menstruation, usually between 45 and 50. The experience can be very disturbing emotionally and physically, but it does not last long and does not result in any permanent loss of sexual desire.

Menstruation: The discharge of unneeded tissue and blood from the womb through the vagina at approximately monthly intervals except during pregnancy. From the Latin word meaning "month."

Miscarriage: The accidental termination of pregnancy before the embryo or fetus can survive independently. Usually caused by exhaustion, injury, disease, or malformation of the embryo.

Mons Veneris: The triangular mound of fat just above the female vulva. From the Latin meaning "mount of love."

Narcissism: Love of oneself or one's own body. From the story of the Greek youth Narcissus who fell in love with his own reflection in the water.

Necking: Generally, fondling or kissing of the body above the waist.

Nocturnal Emission: An involuntary ejaculation of semen during sleep or on awakening. Commonly called a "wet dream."

Nucleus: The center or core of a cell, which contains the chromosomes, which carry hereditary characteristics.

Nymphomania: The condition of a woman who is unable to achieve sexual satisfaction, and desires continuously repeated experiences. Usually psychological in origin, but occasionally due to physical causes. Literally "beauty-madness."

Obscene: Disgusting or revolting. In legal terminology "tending to corrupt or deprave."

Oedipus Complex: Freud's term for the unconscious force which leads the infant to desire the parent of the other sex and envy the parent of its own sex. Taken from the Greek story of Oedipus who killed his father and married his mother, not knowing who they were.

Onanism: Masturbation. From the (incorrect) tradition that the condemnation of Onan in the Bible was due to his practicing masturbation.

Oral-Genital: Stimulation of the genitals by the mouth; for which the terms *cunnilingus* or *fellatio* are sometimes used.

Orgasm: The climax of sexual arousal in which nervous and muscular tension is released in highly pleasurable physical spasms. From the Greek word meaning "to be excited."

Ovaries: The two organs, located on either side of the uterus, in which female sex cells or ova are stored. Each ovary is about two inches long, an inch wide, and a quarter of an inch thick. They also produce certain essential female hormones. Literally "belonging to the eggs."

Ovulation: The process by which approximately every month one ovum is released from an ovary from puberty until the menopause.

Ovum: The female sex cell. From the Latin word for "egg."

Pedophilia: A condition in which an adult male seeks sexual contact with a child. Although a criminal offense such behavior does not usually involve violence or actual

intercourse. From the Latin meaning "lover of children."
Peeping Tom: An adult male who obsessively seeks sexual satisfaction through observing women undressing or naked (in private). A voyeur.
Penis: The male sex organ through which semen and sperm are ejected and urine passed. From the Latin word originally meaning "tail."
Perversion: Strictly "a distortion of original purpose," but commonly any condition of (sexual) abnormality which is disapproved or illegal.
Petting: Generally, sexual intimacy beyond necking that stops short of intercourse. Heavy petting usually refers to manual contact with the genitals of the partner.
Phallic: Relating to the penis. From the Greek word for the male sex organ.
Pill: An inclusive term for several oral contraceptive drugs which all modify the female hormone balance so that no ripe eggs are released from the ovaries and fertilization cannot take place.
Placenta: A flat spongy structure which grows inside the womb during pregnancy and through which food goes from the mother to the embryo (fetus) via the umbilical cord and waste products pass from the embryo to the mother.
Pornography: The use of books, pictures or entertainment to encourage or arouse sexual desire.
Premature Ejaculation: Ejaculation of sperm and semen before the penis has fully entered the vagina in intercourse. Usually due to emotional causes such as anxiety or shame. Technically called *ejaculatio praecox* (Latin).
Prepuce: See Foreskin.
Promiscuity: Engagement in sexual intimacy, particularly intercourse, on a transient basis without affection or concern for the other person involved. From the Latin meaning "mixing with reduced value."
Prostitute: Someone who indiscriminately offers his or her body at a price for the sexual satisfaction of another person. From the Latin meaning "offer or place in public."

Psychiatry: The treatment of mental or emotional disorders, by physical and/or psychological means. In practice many psychiatrists use a combination of drugs and psychotherapy.
Psychoanalysis: The theory of human behavior and method of treatment for emotional problems devised by Sigmund Freud. One among many forms of psychotherapy.
Psychology: The study of the human mind. From the Greek word for "soul" or "life."
Psychopath: A person who has (or appears to have) no social or moral sense or conscience.
Psychotherapy: The treatment of mental and emotional disorders by psychological (as distinct from physical) means. Psychoanalysis is one of many systems of psychotherapy.
Puberty: The process of becoming physically capable of sexual activity and reproduction. From the Latin for "groin."
Pubic Hair: The hair which begins to grow at puberty on the lower abdomen around the genitals.
Rape: Intercourse with a woman against her will. Rape is a serious offense punishable with severe penalties. If the girl is under a certain age (varying between 14 and 21 according to the state) "statutory rape" is involved even if she consents.
Rhythm Method: Birth control through abstinence from intercourse during the period (between 8 and 16 days in each month) when fertilization is possible.
Sadism: The attainment of sexual pleasure by causing pain or humiliation to the partner. Derived from the Marquis de Sade, an eighteenth century deviant who described his perversions with some literary skill.
Safe Period: The days of the menstrual cycle during which fertilization cannot take place.
Sapphic: See **Lesbian.**
Scrotum: The sack of skin and muscle containing the testicles.
Semen: The sticky whitish fluid in which the sperm are

discharged from the penis during ejaculation. From the Latin meaning "to sow."

Sodomy: A term sometimes used to include several legally forbidden sexual acts, sometimes more precisely for homosexual behavior, or specifically anal sex. Derived (almost certainly mistakenly) from the story of the destruction of the city of Sodom in the Old Testament.

Sperm: The male sex cell, from the Greek spermatozoon (plural spermatozoa) meaning literally "life reproducing."

Sterility: Inability to produce offspring. Usually this term is used when the condition is final, as when the ovaries or testicles have been removed by surgery. When the condition is temporary the term infertility is normally used.

Syphilis: The most serious venereal disease, transmitted by kissing and other contacts as well as through intercourse.

Testicles: The two organs which produce male sperm and hormones, situated in the scrotum. From the Latin "testes."

Transsexual: A person who, while brought up as a member of one sex (usually because possessing the external genitals of that sex), feels that he or she really belongs to the other sex. Some transsexuals are able to change their sexual identification and function as a result of surgery. To be distinguished from a hermaphrodite, homosexual or transvestite.

Transvestite: A person who, while knowing that he or she belongs to one sex, likes to dress and act as a member of the other sex. From the Latin for "change of dress."

Trauma: An experience which has lasting and deleterious effects on the personality.

Umbilical Cord: The ropelike tube connecting the fetus at the navel with the placenta in the womb.

Unconscious: That part of the human self which is not open to direct examination or expression, but which (according to Freud and others) plays a basic role in the development of the personality, primarily as a result of forgotten experiences in childhood.

Urethra: The duct through which urine passes from the

bladder through the penis (in the male) or the vulva (in the female). In the male it also serves as the passage for the discharge of semen in ejaculation.

Uterus: The womb. An organ approximately the size and shape of a pear, in the lower abdomen, in which a baby develops before birth.

Vagina: The primary female sex organ which the penis enters during intercourse and through which menstruation and birth take place. From the Latin "sheath, or scabbard."

Vas Deferens: The duct along which sperm travel from the epididymis to the urethra.

Venereal: Pertaining to sex or the sexual organs, particularly (though not exclusively) diseases such as syphilis and gonorrhea. From the name of the ancient Roman goddess of sensual love, Venus.

Voyeur: See **Peeping Tom.**

Vulva: The external covering of the female sex organs, consisting of two folds, the labia majora and labia minora. From the Latin word meaning "wrap."

Wet Dream: See **Nocturnal Emission.**

Womb: See **Uterus.**

Zygote: The fertilized egg or ovum before it has become attached to the wall of the uterus.

Books for Further Reading

The author of this book, Richard Hettlinger, has written a book for college students, *Sex Isn't That Simple* (New York: Continuum, 1974) which goes into all the subjects discussed here in more depth. Many high-school juniors and seniors read it and find it interests them.

If you want a reliable reference book covering all aspects, James McCary's *Human Sexuality* (New York: Van Nostrand, 1973) is highly recommended.

On specific issues these books are helpful:

REPRODUCTION AND BIRTH

A Child is Born—The Drama of Life Before Birth by A. Lennart Nilsson (New York: Delacorte, 1977). Remarkable photographs of a live embryo in the womb.

Facts About Sex for Today's Youth by Sol Gordon (New York: Lippincott & Crowell, 1973). Good, clear illustrations of the growth of the fetus and the process of birth.

PUBERTY

"What's Happening to Me?" by Peter Mayle (Seacaucus, N.J.: Lyle Stuart, 1975). A straightforward guide to help preadolescents.

Growing Up—'Specially for Pre-Teens and Young Teens by Marilyn Lyman (Planned Parenthood Center of Syra-

130

CAMROSE LUTHERAN COLLEGE LIBRARY

HQ
35
H45

cuse). Fourteen illustrated pages on menstruation, wet dreams, masturbation and conception.

DATING

You Would if You Loved Me by Sol Gordon (New York: Bantam Books, 1978). A witty collection of the "lines" boys use and suggestions for answering them.

Sex and Sensibility: A New Look at Being a Woman by Elizabeth Whelan (New York: McGraw-Hill, 1974) and *Making Sense Out of Sex: A New Look at Being a Man* by Stephen and Elizabeth Whelan (New York: McGraw-Hill, 1975) are helpful in understanding the emotional aspects of getting to know oneself and the other sex.

LOVE AND SEX

Love and Sex in Plain Language by Eric Johnson (New York: Bantam Books, 1979) and *Sex with Love: A Guide for Young People* by Eleanor Hamilton (Boston: Beacon Press, 1978) both emphasize that sex is part of the whole person and encourage its expression in responsible relationships.

BIRTH CONTROL

Sex and Birth Control: A Guide for the Young by E. James Lieberman and Ellen Peck (New York: Schocken Books, 1975) provides full information and encourages the sensible use of contraceptives.

Conception, Birth and Contraception: A Visual Presentation by Robert J. Demarest and John J. Sciarra (New York: McGraw-Hill, 1976). A pictorial presentation of human reproduction and the various methods of birth control.

VENEREAL DISEASES

Facts About VD for Today's Youth by Sol Gordon (New York: Lippincott & Crowell, 1973). An illustrated explanation of the symptoms, consequences, and cure of venereal diseases.

132   *Growing Up with Sex*

PREGNANCY AND PARENTHOOD

Only Human: Teenage Pregnancy by Marion Howard (New
York: Continuum, 1975).

Parenting: A Guide for Young People by Sol Gordon and
Mina Wollin (New York: Sadlier, 1975). A helpful
book for potential parents.

ABORTION

Abortion: The Agonizing Decision by David R. Mace (Nash-
ville: Abingdon, 1972). Presents the alternatives
clearly and objectively.